SMALL BUBBLE, BIG IMPACT

DR. SREERAJ GOPI, PhD, FRSC

notionpress.com

INDIA • SINGAPORE • MALAYSIA

ISBN
Paperback 979-8-90451-357-3
Hardcase 979-8-90479-285-5

Contents

Chapter 01

Why We Need to Talk About Liposomes

The word "liposome" has recently taken a curious journey from the pages of pharmaceutical textbooks into the everyday conversations of health-conscious consumers. Not long ago, if you mentioned liposomes at a dinner party, you'd probably be met with puzzled stares or a polite change of topic. Today, however, especially among people who regularly take vitamins, herbal extracts, or nutritional supplements, the term is not only familiar but even fashionable.

Part of this shift can be traced to an unexpected source: a global pandemic. The COVID-19 crisis not only altered the way we work, travel, and interact—it also catapulted certain scientific terms into the public spotlight. Among them were mRNA, spike protein, and yes, liposome. Both Moderna and Pfizer–BioNTech, the pharmaceutical giants behind two of the first COVID-19 vaccines, used liposome-like nanostructures—more specifically, lipid nanoparticles—to protect and deliver fragile strands of mRNA into human cells. Overnight, millions of people became vaguely aware that these tiny fat-based spheres were critical to the success of these groundbreaking vaccines.

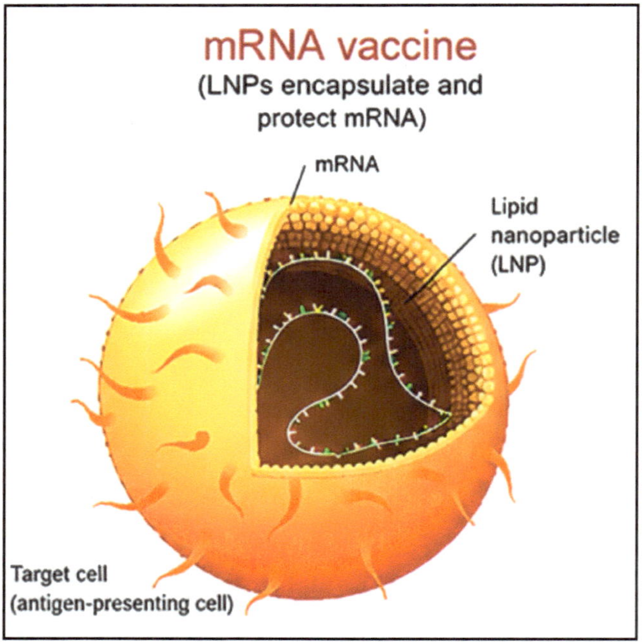

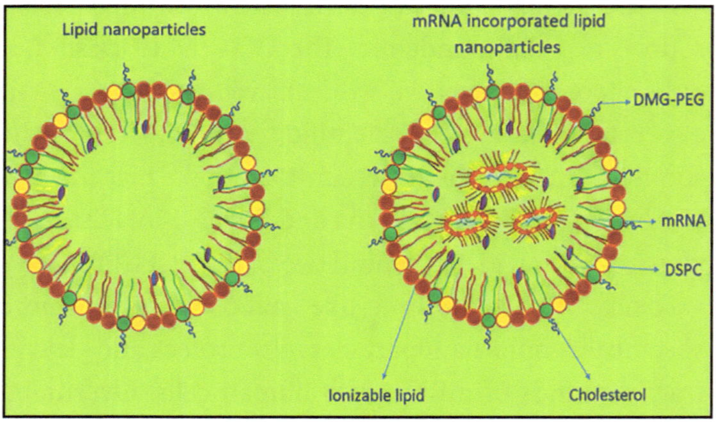

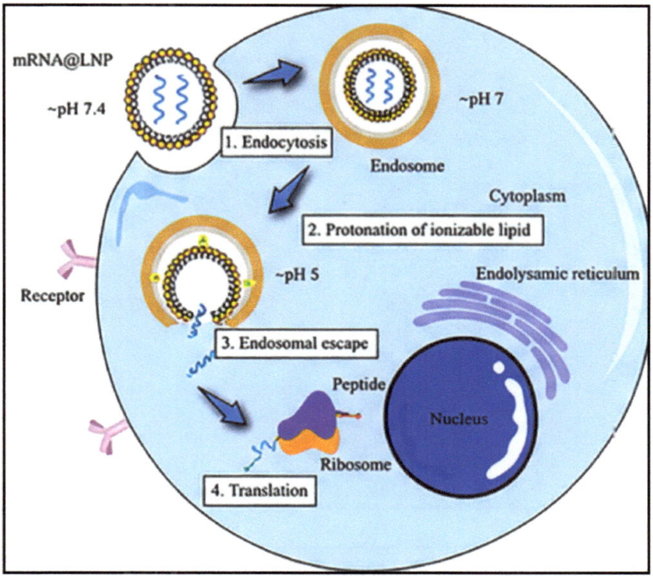
mRNA@LNP
~pH 7.4
~pH 7
1. Endocytosis
Endosome
Cytoplasm
2. Protonation of ionizable lipid
~pH 5
Endolysamic reticulum
Receptor
3. Endosomal escape
Peptide
Nucleus
Ribosome
4. Translation

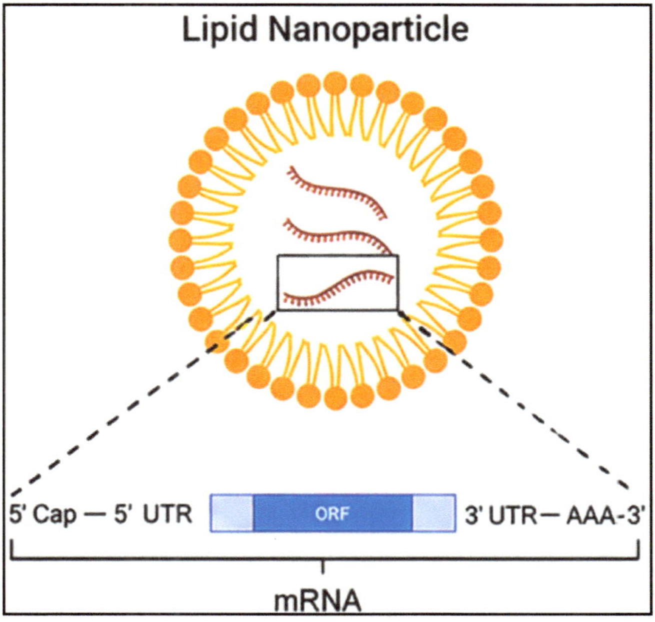
Lipid Nanoparticle
5' Cap — 5' UTR
ORF
3' UTR— AAA-3'
mRNA

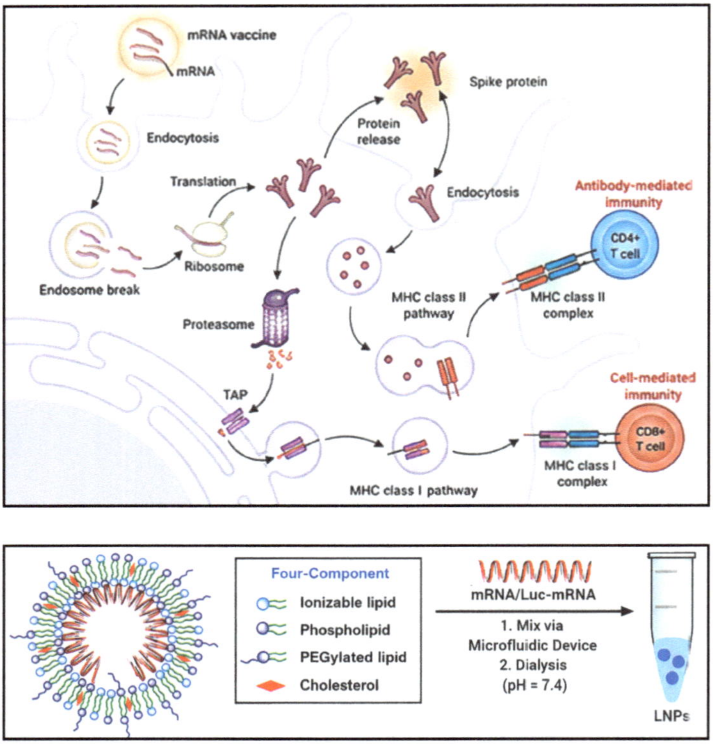

Figure 1. Lipid nanoparticles for mRNA delivery.

Schematic representation of lipid nanoparticle (LNP) structure, composition, and mechanism of action. LNPs encapsulate mRNA within a lipid matrix composed of ionizable lipids, phospholipids, cholesterol, and PEGylated lipids. Following administration, LNPs are internalized by cells via endocytosis, escape from endosomes, and release mRNA into the cytoplasm, where it is translated into protein, enabling therapeutic or immunological effects.

But this is only part of the story. Long before they were deployed against a novel coronavirus, liposomes had been studied for decades in pharmaceutical research labs. They are not magical new inventions; rather, they are the elegant product of years of experimentation and refinement in the quest for better drug delivery systems. And now, as supplement companies in the West increasingly market liposomal vitamin C, liposomal glutathione, and other liposome-encased nutrients, the term has jumped from the scientific literature to product labels at your local health store.

In the coming chapters, this book will be entirely devoted to exploring liposomes—what they are, why they matter, and how they are changing the way we think about medicine and nutrition. But before we dive into these microscopic marvels, it's important to first understand what happens to a medicine or supplement after you swallow it.

Why? Because without this context, the significance of liposomes might be lost. To truly appreciate why pharmaceutical scientists went to such lengths to develop liposomal delivery systems, you need to know the "obstacles course" that every pill, capsule, or powder must navigate inside your body before it can do you any good.

Chapter

02

The Fate of a Medicine – An Obstacle Course Inside the Body

When you pop a vitamin C tablet into your mouth, or swallow an antibiotic capsule with a glass of water, it feels like a simple act. The reality, however, is anything but simple. That tablet is about to embark on an intricate, hazardous journey through the hostile landscapes of your digestive system. Only a fraction of what you ingest may actually reach the cells where it's needed.

Let's follow this journey step by step.

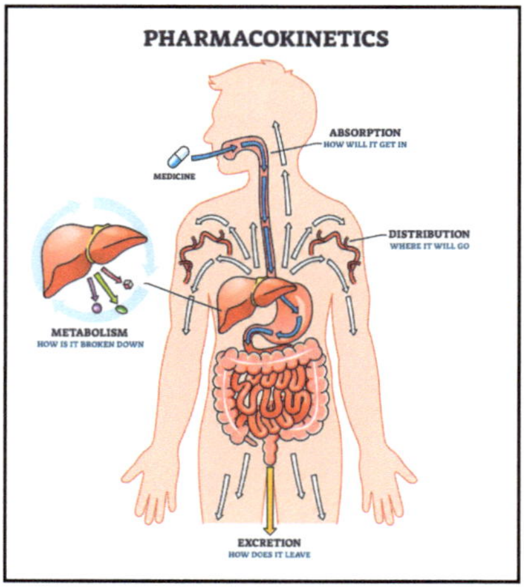

Figure 2. Pharmacokinetics of an orally administered drug (ADME).

Illustration of drug absorption from the gastrointestinal tract, distribution via systemic circulation, metabolism primarily in the liver (including first-pass effect), and elimination through excretory pathways.

2.1. From Pill to Cell: The Journey of a Medicine Inside Your Body

2.1.1. Entry – The Mouth and the First Contact

When a patient swallows a medicine—be it a tablet, capsule, syrup, or suspension—it embarks on a complex and highly coordinated journey. In the mouth, the main purpose is mechanical breakdown (chewing) and partial dissolution in saliva. While most drugs are not significantly absorbed here, a few exceptions like nitroglycerin (for angina) can be taken sublingually for rapid absorption through oral mucosa.

Saliva pH: Around 6.5–7.5, slightly acidic to neutral, which means most solid dosage forms remain intact and are simply carried down the esophagus.

2.1.2. The Stomach – The Acidic Fortress

Once a medicine is swallowed, it enters the stomach—a muscular, dynamic chamber designed to break down food. For a drug, however, this environment can be both a gateway and a barrier. The stomach is filled with gastric fluid containing hydrochloric acid, making it one of the most chemically aggressive regions in the body. When the stomach is empty, the acidity is extremely high, with a pH ranging from about 1.5 to 2.0. After a meal, this acidity is partially reduced, rising to around pH 3.0 to 5.0 as food temporarily buffers the acid. Even in this "less acidic" state, the environment remains harsh enough to challenge many delicate molecules.

This acidic setting plays a crucial role in determining the fate of a medicine. Some drugs are inherently unstable in low pH and begin to degrade before they can be absorbed. A classic example is Omeprazole, which is highly sensitive to stomach acid. To protect such drugs, scientists design special coatings—known as enteric coatings—that remain intact in the stomach and dissolve only after reaching the more neutral environment of the small intestine.

The chemistry of the drug itself also influences how it behaves in the stomach. Weakly acidic drugs, such as Aspirin, tend to remain in an uncharged form in this acidic environment. In this state, they can pass through biological membranes more easily, allowing a limited degree of absorption directly from the stomach lining. However, the overall surface area of the stomach is relatively small compared to the intestine, so this absorption is modest. In contrast, weakly basic drugs like Morphine become ionized in the acidic gastric environment. Once ionized, they struggle to cross cell membranes and are therefore poorly absorbed at this stage.

Beyond its chemical effects, the stomach also exerts a strong physical influence on the medicine. Through rhythmic contractions, it churns and mixes its contents, breaking tablets and capsules into smaller fragments. This mechanical action increases the surface area of the drug, allowing it to dissolve more efficiently in the gastric fluid. Dissolution is a critical step, because only dissolved molecules can be absorbed further along the digestive tract.

In essence, the stomach acts as both a testing ground and a gatekeeper. It determines which molecules can survive, which begin to dissolve, and which must be protected to continue their journey. For many drugs, passing through this acidic fortress intact is the first major challenge in reaching their ultimate destination within the body.

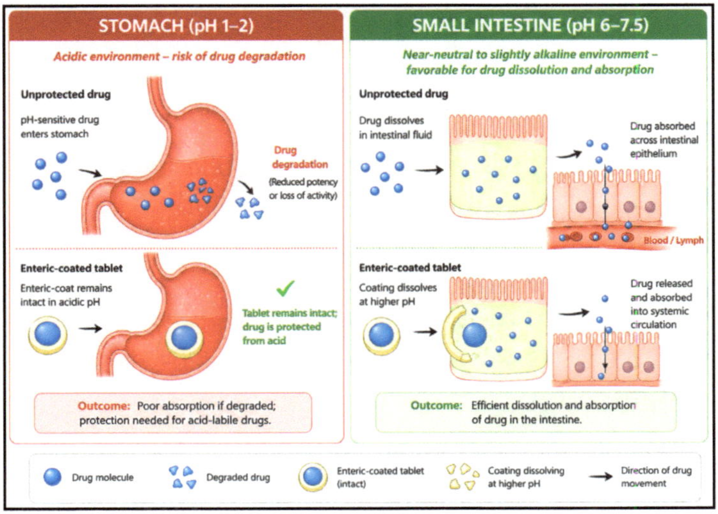

Figure 3. Effect of gastrointestinal pH on drug stability and release.

Schematic comparison of drug behavior in the acidic stomach environment (pH 1–2), where pH-sensitive drugs may degrade, and the near-neutral to slightly alkaline small intestine (pH 6–7.5), where drugs dissolve and are absorbed. Enteric coating is illustrated as a protective strategy that prevents drug degradation in the stomach and enables release in the intestine.

2.1.3. The Small Intestine – The Main Absorption Highway

From the stomach, the medicine passes through the pyloric sphincter into the duodenum, the first part of the small intestine.

pH Transition:

Duodenum: ~6.0

Jejunum: ~6.5–7.0

Ileum: ~7.4

The sharp rise in pH comes from bile and pancreatic secretions neutralizing stomach acid.

Why the small intestine is the major absorption site:

Huge surface area—thanks to villi and microvilli, the intestine's surface area can reach 200–300 m^2 (like a tennis court).

Rich blood supply—absorbed drug molecules quickly enter the portal circulation.

Long transit time—medicines spend hours here, maximizing absorption opportunities.

Optimal pH for most drugs—many are unionized and lipid-soluble here.

Absorption mechanisms:

Once a medicine reaches the small intestine and dissolves in the surrounding fluid, it faces its most important challenge: crossing the intestinal wall to enter the bloodstream. This wall is not simply a passive barrier. It is a living, highly selective membrane that decides what enters the body and what stays behind. To pass through it, drug molecules rely on a few fundamental transport mechanisms. Each pathway reflects a different strategy—some simple and effortless, others highly controlled and energy-driven.

The most common pathway is **passive diffusion**, a process guided by nothing more than natural movement. Molecules tend to move from areas where they are abundant to areas where they are less concentrated, much like a drop of ink spreading through water. Small, lipid-soluble drugs take advantage of this. Because the intestinal cell membrane is made of lipids, these molecules can slip through it with relative ease. Drugs such as Ibuprofen and diazepam move across the membrane in this way. No energy is required, no assistance is needed—the molecule simply follows its concentration gradient. The more lipophilic and smaller the molecule, the easier this journey becomes. This is why many drugs are chemically designed to have some degree of fat solubility.

However, not all molecules are able to pass so freely. Many drugs are too polar or too large to dissolve in the lipid membrane. For these, the body provides an alternative route known as **facilitated diffusion**. In this mechanism, specialized proteins embedded in the cell membrane act as carriers. These carriers recognize certain molecular shapes and allow them to pass through, almost like a revolving door that opens only for specific guests. The process still follows a concentration gradient—moving from high to low concentration—but requires the presence of these transport proteins. Some vitamins and drug-like molecules use this pathway when their structure resembles naturally occurring compounds that the body is accustomed to transporting.

A more controlled and energy-dependent mechanism is **active transport**. Here, the body actively pulls molecules across the membrane, often against their concentration gradient. This means that even if there is already a higher concentration of the molecule inside the cell, the transport system can still move more of it inward. This process requires energy, usually in the form of ATP, and relies on highly specific transporter proteins. A classic example is Levodopa, a drug used in Parkinson's disease. Levodopa closely resembles amino acids, and the body's amino acid transporters mistakenly recognize it as a nutrient and carry it across the intestinal wall. This clever mimicry allows the drug to take advantage of the body's own nutrient absorption systems.

For larger and more complex molecules, such as certain peptides and proteins, even these transport systems are not sufficient. In such cases, the body employs a process called **endocytosis**. This is a more elaborate mechanism in which the cell membrane wraps around the molecule, forming a small vesicle that pulls it inside the cell. It is as if the cell briefly engulfs the molecule to bring it in. While this pathway is less common for most conventional drugs, it becomes important for larger biological molecules, including some therapeutic peptides and nanoparticles. It is also one of the mechanisms through which advanced delivery systems, such as liposomes, can enter cells.

Together, these four pathways—passive diffusion, facilitated diffusion, active transport, and endocytosis—form the fundamental routes by which medicines move from the intestine into the body. Each drug, depending on its size, structure, and chemical nature, finds its own preferred path. Understanding these pathways is essential, because the success of a medicine does not depend only on its chemical activity, but also on its ability to cross this biological barrier and reach its target.

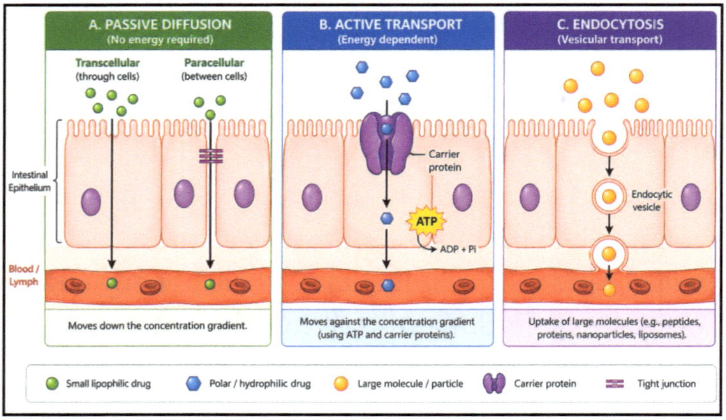

Figure 4. Mechanisms of drug absorption across the intestinal epithelium.

Schematic illustration of the primary pathways of drug transport across the intestinal barrier, including passive diffusion (transcellular and paracellular movement down a concentration gradient), carrier-mediated active transport requiring energy, and endocytosis for the uptake of larger molecules such as peptides, proteins, and nanoparticles.

Chapter

03

First-Pass Effect – The Liver's Checkpoint

After a drug is absorbed from the small intestine, it does not immediately enter the general bloodstream. Instead, it is first directed through a specialized vascular route known as the hepatic portal vein, which delivers it straight to the liver. This journey is remarkably fast. In most cases, dissolved drug molecules begin to reach the liver **within a few minutes of intestinal absorption—typically around 2 to 5 minutes**, depending on factors such as gastric emptying, intestinal motility, and blood flow. Under fed conditions, or with slow-release formulations, this time may extend to **10–30 minutes**, but the liver remains the first major organ encountered.

The liver functions as a biochemical checkpoint, carefully processing incoming substances before they are allowed to circulate throughout the body. Within liver cells, a sophisticated system of enzymes—particularly those of the cytochrome P450 family—modifies drug molecules through reactions such as oxidation, reduction, and hydrolysis.

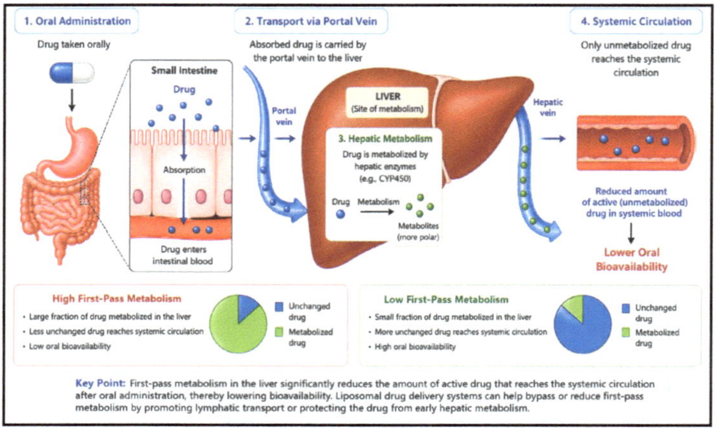

Figure 5. First-pass metabolism and its impact on oral drug bioavailability.

Schematic representation of the first-pass effect, where a drug absorbed from the small intestine is transported to the liver via the portal vein and undergoes metabolic transformation before reaching systemic circulation. This process reduces the amount of active drug available, thereby decreasing oral bioavailability.

This transformation can have different outcomes. Some drugs are partially or completely inactivated during this stage, reducing the amount that ultimately reaches the bloodstream. Others are activated here. Certain medicines are deliberately designed as inactive precursors, known as prodrugs, which rely on liver metabolism to become therapeutically active. A well-known example is Codeine, which is converted into morphine after hepatic processing.

This phenomenon, known as the **first-pass effect**, plays a decisive role in determining bioavailability. Drugs such as Propranolol undergo significant first-pass metabolism, meaning only a fraction of the administered dose reaches systemic circulation. In contrast, drugs like Nitroglycerin are so extensively metabolized in the liver that oral administration becomes ineffective, necessitating alternative routes such as sublingual delivery.

In essence, the liver acts as both a filter and a regulator—reducing toxicity, activating certain drugs, and determining how much of a substance is allowed to proceed further into the body.

Chapter

04

Systemic Circulation – The Highway to the Cells

Once a drug passes through the liver and survives initial metabolism, it enters the systemic circulation—the vast network of blood vessels that distributes it throughout the body. At this stage, the drug is carried like a passenger on a dynamic and highly organized transport system.

Distribution is influenced primarily by blood flow. Organs such as the brain, heart, liver, and kidneys receive a disproportionately large share of cardiac output, and therefore encounter the drug earlier and in higher concentrations. Tissues with lower blood flow, such as muscle or fat, are reached more slowly.

At the same time, a significant portion of the drug may bind to plasma proteins. Acidic drugs tend to associate with albumin, while basic drugs often bind to globulins. This binding is reversible and creates a reservoir of drug in the bloodstream. Only the unbound fraction remains free to cross membranes and exert pharmacological action, while the bound fraction serves as a slowly available reserve.

The ability of a drug to leave the bloodstream and enter tissues depends on its physicochemical properties. Lipid-soluble molecules diffuse readily across cell membranes, moving into tissues with minimal resistance. In contrast, hydrophilic molecules rely on transport proteins or aqueous channels to traverse these barriers. As a result, even within systemic circulation, the chemical nature of the drug continues to dictate its journey.

4.1. Cellular Entry – The Final Frontier

Reaching a tissue does not guarantee therapeutic action. For most drugs, the true site of action lies within the cell, making the cell membrane the final and often decisive barrier.

This membrane, composed of a lipid bilayer, selectively permits entry based on molecular properties. Lipophilic drugs dissolve in the membrane and pass through by passive diffusion, often with remarkable efficiency. Many small-molecule drugs rely on this mechanism.

Hydrophilic compounds, however, face a more restricted pathway. They may depend on membrane transporters or specialized entry mechanisms to gain access. In certain cases, the cell actively engulfs the drug through processes such as endocytosis, enclosing it within vesicles before releasing it internally.

The success of this step determines whether the drug can interact with its intended target—be it an enzyme, receptor, or intracellular structure. A molecule that fails to cross the membrane remains pharmacologically ineffective, regardless of its intrinsic potency.

Chapter

05

Metabolism – The Body's Detoxification System

After a drug has exerted its therapeutic effect, the body initiates processes to remove it. This is achieved through metabolism, a series of enzymatic reactions that convert the drug into more water-soluble forms suitable for elimination.

The liver remains the primary site for this transformation, although other tissues such as the intestine, kidneys, and lungs may also contribute. Drug metabolism generally occurs in two phases.

In **Phase I reactions**, the molecule undergoes chemical modification through oxidation, reduction, or hydrolysis, often mediated by cytochrome P450 enzymes. These reactions introduce or expose functional groups, increasing the molecule's polarity.

In **Phase II reactions**, the drug or its Phase I metabolite is conjugated with endogenous substances such as glucuronic acid, sulfate, or glutathione. This step significantly enhances water solubility, facilitating excretion through urine or bile.

Metabolism may inactivate the drug, generate active metabolites, or occasionally produce toxic intermediates. Regardless of the outcome, the process reflects the body's continuous effort to maintain balance—transforming foreign molecules into forms that can be safely removed.

Two Phases of Metabolism:

Phase I (Functionalization): Oxidation, reduction, hydrolysis—usually by cytochrome P450 enzymes. Makes drug more polar.

Phase II (Conjugation): Attachment of a polar group (e.g., glucuronic acid, sulfate) to make it water-soluble.

Some drugs are excreted unchanged (e.g., aminoglycosides), but most are metabolized before leaving the body.

5.1. Elimination – The Exit Routes

The main ways drugs leave the body:

Kidneys (urine)—the most common route; depends on filtration, secretion, and reabsorption.

Bile (feces)—large, polar metabolites are excreted into bile and leave via feces.

Lungs (exhalation)—important for volatile drugs like anesthetics.

Sweat, saliva, tears, breast milk—minor routes, but important in special contexts.

Renal elimination steps:

Glomerular filtration—small molecules filtered into urine

Tubular secretion—active pumping of drug into tubules

Tubular reabsorption—lipid-soluble drugs may be reabsorbed into blood

This intricate journey ensures that only a fraction of what we swallow reaches the site of action—but with clever formulation, dosing, and delivery systems, we can make medicines more efficient, targeted, and safe.

5.2. A Morning Pill and the Lesson It Teaches

Every morning, millions of people around the world wake up and reach for a tiny tablet—**thyroxine**, or *levothyroxine sodium*. It's one of the most prescribed medicines on Earth, used to treat **hypothyroidism**, a condition where the thyroid gland doesn't produce enough hormones to keep the body's metabolism running smoothly.

The pill itself looks harmless—small, white, almost weightless. But its journey inside the body is anything but simple. Thyroxine has to be **absorbed in the small intestine**, mostly in the **duodenum and upper jejunum**. The problem is that its absorption is easily disturbed—by food, coffee, minerals like calcium and iron, even by the pH and fiber content of breakfast.

When a patient swallows thyroxine with food, its bioavailability drops drastically—sometimes from 80% down to less than 40%. The drug molecules get trapped, bound, or degraded before they can even cross the intestinal wall. And since the thyroid hormone system is extremely sensitive, even small fluctuations in absorption can upset the delicate hormonal balance.

That's why doctors insist that **thyroxine must be taken on an empty stomach—ideally 2 to 3 hours before eating or at least 30 to 60 minutes before breakfast**. It's not superstition; it's *pharmaceutical physics*. The stomach must be calm and empty so the tablet can dissolve in a predictable environment. When taken with food, proteins and fibers compete for absorption sites, and minerals form insoluble complexes that trap the drug.

Interestingly, thyroxine is also a great example of how the *timing of delivery* can define a drug's success. The same molecule, taken at the wrong time, behaves almost like a different drug. This shows why scientists are so obsessed with "delivery"—not just the molecule itself, but *how, when, and where* it reaches its target.

Imagine, then, if we could design a system that protects thyroxine as it travels through the stomach, releases it exactly in the small intestine, and ensures consistent absorption every day—that's what **drug delivery systems** try to achieve.

So, every time someone patiently waits before breakfast to take their thyroid pill, they are unknowingly practicing one of the fundamental lessons of modern pharmaceutics: It's not just what you take that matters, but how you deliver it.

Chapter

06

From Ancient Healing to Liposomes – The Journey of Drug Delivery

Imagine you have a precious gift to send to a friend who lives far away. The gift is fragile, expensive, and must arrive in perfect condition—at exactly the right time. You wouldn't just toss it into the post without protection, right? You'd wrap it carefully, choose a reliable courier, and maybe even add a note with delivery instructions.

Now, replace that "gift" with a life-saving medicine inside your body. When a doctor prescribes a drug, the challenge is not only getting it into your system, but also ensuring it reaches the exact place where it's needed, in the right amount, at the right time—without being destroyed or causing harm along the way. This is what scientists call **drug delivery**.

The human body is both a wonderland and a battlefield for medicines. Stomach acid, enzymes, and liver metabolism act like strict security guards—breaking down many drugs before they ever reach their targets. Even if a drug survives, it might wander aimlessly throughout the body instead of going straight to the problem area, leading to side effects.

To solve this, scientists create *drug delivery systems*—like intelligent couriers that protect the medicine, guide it safely through the body, and release it precisely where it's needed.

If that still sounds abstract, think about how we launch satellites into space. A satellite is like the **drug**—valuable, full of purpose, but powerless on its own. It cannot reach its orbit without help. That's where the **rocket** comes in—it provides the thrust, protection, and direction to place the satellite exactly where it belongs. Once the rocket completes its job, the satellite begins to work, sending signals or capturing images from orbit.

In the same way, a drug delivery system acts like the rocket—it carries the drug (the satellite) safely through the harsh journey of the body, protecting it from destruction and releasing it precisely at the target site. Without the rocket, the satellite is useless. And without an efficient delivery system, even the most powerful drug may never fulfill its purpose.

Before modern science, people didn't talk about "drug delivery systems," but they were still trying to solve the same problem—how to make medicines more effective and less harmful. That story began thousands of years ago.

6.1. Ancient Roots of Medicine Delivery

The need to control how medicines enter the body is as old as medicine itself. Let's take a trip through history.

6.1.1. Ancient Greece: Wrapping Nature in Nature

In the time of Hippocrates (around 400 BCE), Greek healers understood that some medicines were too strong to give directly. They wrapped plant extracts in honey, wax, or dough—not just for taste but to mask bitterness, reduce stomach irritation, and control release. Honey wasn't just a sweetener—it had antimicrobial properties and protected delicate herbal components.

Greek physicians also used ointments and balms to deliver medicines through the skin. Olive oil mixed with crushed herbs allowed slow absorption into the body, much like today's transdermal patches.

6.1.2. Ancient India: Ayurveda and the Art of Formulation

Ayurveda, India's traditional system of medicine (dating back over 3,000 years), had a deep understanding of drug delivery, even without modern terminology. Ayurvedic practitioners classified medicines into different dosage forms:

Kashayam (herbal decoctions) for fast action

Lehyam (herbal jams) with jaggery or honey for sustained release

Ghee-based preparations (Ghrita) for carrying fat-soluble compounds into tissues

Bhasma (calcined minerals) for slow, long-lasting effects

The choice of form depended on how fast the medicine needed to work, how long it should last, and which part of the body it should reach. Ghee, for example, could carry certain herbal molecules deep into tissues, much like a primitive lipid-based delivery system.

6.1.3. Ghee-Based Delivery Systems—The Ancient Lipid Carriers

Among the many ingenious dosage forms in Ayurveda, none illustrates the art of drug delivery more beautifully than **Ghrita**, the ghee-based formulation. While ancient physicians saw it as a sacred, nourishing medium, modern science recognizes it as a **biocompatible lipid vehicle**—an early prototype of what we now call **lipid-based drug delivery systems (LBDDS)**.

In Ghrita, fats were not merely flavoring or binding agents—they were **functional carriers** designed to transport herbal molecules deep into the body, protect them from degradation, and ensure sustained, targeted action.

6.1.4. The Science Behind the Tradition

Ghee (clarified butter) is primarily composed of **triglycerides, phospholipids, cholesterol, and minor bioactive lipids**. When used in formulations, it creates a **lipophilic microenvironment** that dissolves nonpolar phytoconstituents—alkaloids, terpenoids, flavonoids, and essential oils—enhancing their bioavailability and cellular uptake.

From a modern chemical perspective, the ghee matrix behaves like a **micro-emulsion or lipid vesicle precursor**. When mixed with aqueous or semi-aqueous herbal extracts under controlled heat (a process described in Ayurveda as *Sneha Paka*), amphiphilic molecules from both the herbs and the ghee form **colloidal dispersions**, stabilized by natural phospholipids and minor emulsifiers present in milk fat.

These colloidal droplets, though never intentionally nano-sized in ancient times, share functional similarities with **liposomes**, **niosomes**, and **self-emulsifying lipid systems**. The lipid phase encapsulates hydrophobic compounds, while certain glycosides and polar phenolics remain interfacially associated, creating a spectrum of solubility states that together enhance absorption across intestinal membranes.

6.2. Physicochemical Dynamics – How Ghee Mimics Modern Carriers

When heated with aqueous decoctions (*Kashayam*), ghee undergoes **partial emulsification**. The process involves:

1. **Phase inversion and vesiculation**—The constant churning and heating under *madhyama agni* (moderate heat) cause microdroplet formation. Fat globules acquire amphiphilic boundaries due to the adsorption of herbal saponins and phospholipids, forming vesicle-like structures.

2. **Interfacial adsorption of actives**—Polar phytochemicals align at the oil-water interface, anchored by hydrogen bonds and hydrophobic interactions. This creates a **diffusion barrier** that slows oxidation and thermal degradation.
3. **Entrapment and partitioning**—Lipophilic molecules (e.g., curcuminoids, boswellic acids, asarones) dissolve directly into the triglyceride core, while intermediate polarity compounds occupy the interface. The result is a **multi-layered encapsulation system** remarkably similar to a modern self-emulsifying drug delivery system (SEDDS).
4. **Solid lipid structuring on cooling**—As the mixture cools, triglycerides re-solidify into a semi-crystalline matrix, trapping actives within ordered lipid lamellae. This slows release and enhances stability—essentially creating a **natural solid-lipid matrix**.

Under microscopic examination, Ghrita-based formulations show **heterogeneous lipid lamellae and vesicular inclusions**—reminiscent of microemulsions and liposomal dispersions described centuries later.

6.3. Gastrointestinal Fate – The Lipid Pathway to Bioavailability

Ayurveda describes ghee (Ghrita) as a substance that can carry medicines deep into the body, nourishing and reaching all tissues (*Dhatus*). While this idea was originally expressed in experiential language, modern pharmacokinetics provides a clear biochemical explanation for this phenomenon. When examined carefully, ghee behaves as a highly effective lipid-based delivery system, closely resembling the strategies used today to improve the absorption of poorly soluble drugs.

After ingestion, ghee enters the digestive tract as a complex mixture of triglycerides, phospholipids, cholesterol, and minor lipid-soluble components. Its transformation begins in the small intestine, where bile salts—natural surfactants secreted by the liver—break down large fat droplets into much smaller emulsified particles. At the same time, pancreatic lipases enzymatically hydrolyze triglycerides into free fatty acids and monoglycerides.

This combination of emulsification and enzymatic digestion leads to the formation of **mixed micelles**—nanoscale aggregates composed of bile salts, fatty acids, phospholipids, and cholesterol. These micelles serve as transport vehicles for lipophilic compounds. Herbal actives that are otherwise poorly soluble in water—such as curcuminoids, carotenoids, or fat-soluble vitamins—readily dissolve into the hydrophobic core of these structures. In effect, the lipid environment created by ghee transforms insoluble molecules into bioavailable forms.

These micelles diffuse through the intestinal fluid and reach the surface of enterocytes, the absorptive cells lining the intestine. At this interface, the lipophilic molecules partition into the cell membrane and enter the cell, primarily through passive diffusion, although certain fractions may also be taken up via endocytosis.

Inside the enterocyte, a critical transformation occurs. The absorbed lipids and associated compounds are reassembled into large, structured particles known as **chylomicrons**. These are specialized lipid transport vehicles composed of triglycerides, phospholipids, cholesterol esters, and apolipoproteins. Their role is to transport dietary lipids efficiently throughout the body.

Here lies the most crucial pharmacokinetic advantage. Unlike water-soluble drugs, which are transported directly from the intestine to the liver via the hepatic portal vein, chylomicrons follow a completely different route. They are released from the enterocytes into the **lymphatic system**, a network of vessels that eventually drains into the systemic circulation through the thoracic duct.

This means that the absorbed compounds **initially bypass the hepatic portal vein and avoid immediate exposure to liver metabolism**.

This phenomenon has been extensively validated in modern pharmacokinetics and is known as **lymphatic transport of lipophilic compounds**. Scientific studies have shown that highly lipophilic molecules (typically with a log P greater than ~5 and significant triglyceride solubility) are preferentially incorporated into chylomicrons and transported via the lymphatic system. This pathway allows them to enter systemic circulation before encountering hepatic enzymes, thereby avoiding or significantly reducing first-pass metabolism.

A classic example of this principle is the immunosuppressant Cyclosporine. When formulated in lipid-based systems, cyclosporine demonstrates enhanced lymphatic transport and improved bioavailability. Similarly, highly lipophilic compounds such as Halofantrine and fat-soluble vitamins show increased systemic exposure when delivered with dietary lipids. Modern drug delivery technologies such as self-emulsifying drug delivery systems (SEDDS) are specifically designed to exploit this pathway.

By bypassing the liver in the early phase, a greater fraction of the active compound remains intact, leading to **higher bioavailability, reduced metabolic loss, and prolonged circulation time**. Only after entering systemic circulation do these compounds gradually reach the liver for metabolism.

In essence, the sequence—lipid digestion, micelle formation, cellular uptake, chylomicron assembly, and lymphatic transport—forms a highly efficient biological pathway for delivering lipophilic molecules. This same pathway is deliberately engineered in modern pharmaceutical systems to enhance the performance of drugs that would otherwise be poorly absorbed or rapidly metabolized.

From a biochemical standpoint, the Ayurvedic concept of ghee "reaching all tissues" can be understood as the combined effect of enhanced solubilization, efficient absorption, lymphatic transport, and improved membrane permeability. Lipids have a natural affinity for biological membranes, which are themselves composed of lipid bilayers. This allows lipid-associated molecules to partition into cell membranes, cross biological barriers, and distribute widely within the body.

Thus, what was once described in metaphorical language aligns closely with well-established scientific principles. Ghee, far from being just a nutritional medium, functions as a **natural lipid delivery system**, capable of enhancing the absorption, distribution, and persistence of bioactive compounds.Top of Form

Bottom of Form

6.4. Molecular Compatibility – Why Herbs Love Ghee

Herbal molecules often pose solubility and stability challenges. Many are **polyphenolic, poorly water-soluble, prone to oxidation**, or unstable in acidic pH. Ghee offers a natural solution:

One of the most fascinating aspects of ghee-based formulations lies in how different classes of herbal compounds interact with the lipid matrix. These interactions are not random; they are governed by the chemical nature of the molecules and the physico-chemical environment created by ghee. When viewed through a modern scientific lens, ghee functions not merely as a carrier but as a multi-phase delivery system, capable of solubilizing, stabilizing, and modulating the release of diverse phytochemicals.

Fat-soluble compounds, particularly terpenoids, find an ideal environment within the triglyceride-rich core of ghee. Molecules such as curcumin from turmeric and shogaols from ginger are highly lipophilic and exhibit very poor solubility in aqueous environments. When administered alone, their absorption is limited, and they are prone to rapid degradation. In the presence of ghee, however, these molecules dissolve readily within the lipid phase, where they are shielded from hydrolytic and oxidative stress. This solubilization significantly enhances their apparent solubility in the gastrointestinal tract, facilitating their incorporation into mixed micelles during digestion. Numerous pharmacokinetic studies have demonstrated that curcumin exhibits markedly improved bioavailability when co-administered with dietary lipids, including ghee or similar fat sources, owing to enhanced micellar solubilization and lymphatic uptake.

Polyphenolic compounds, including flavonoids and tannins, present a more complex behavior. These molecules are amphiphilic in nature—they possess both hydrophilic and hydrophobic regions. Within a ghee-based system, such compounds tend to localize at the oil–water interface, where they can interact simultaneously with lipid components and aqueous phases. This interfacial positioning is of particular importance. It creates a diffusion barrier that slows the release of the compound, effectively resulting in a form of controlled or sustained release. For example, quercetin and catechins have been shown to associate with lipid interfaces, where hydrogen bonding and π–π interactions stabilize their position. This not only moderates their release but also protects them from rapid degradation in the gastrointestinal environment.

Alkaloids and glycosides, which often exhibit intermediate polarity, interact with ghee through a combination of interfacial adsorption and molecular association with phospholipids. Phospholipids naturally present in ghee act as amphiphilic stabilizers, forming microdomains that can accommodate such molecules. Alkaloids like piperine, as well as glycosidic compounds, can associate with these phospholipid-rich regions, enhancing their interaction with biological membranes. This is particularly significant because membrane permeability is a key determinant of absorption. Piperine itself has been widely studied for its ability to enhance the bioavailability of other compounds, partly through its affinity for lipid environments and its effect on membrane dynamics.

Volatile oils, composed largely of small, lipophilic aromatic compounds, benefit from yet another protective mechanism. These compounds are inherently unstable—they evaporate easily and are highly susceptible to oxidation. When incorporated into ghee, they become entrapped within the lipid matrix, reducing their exposure to oxygen and limiting their volatility. Essential oil components such as eugenol, thymol, and menthol demonstrate improved stability when stored in lipid-rich environments. The lipid phase acts as a physical barrier, slowing both evaporation and oxidative degradation, thereby preserving their bioactivity over time.

An equally important, though often overlooked, feature of ghee is its intrinsic antioxidant capacity. Ghee contains naturally occurring antioxidants such as tocopherols (vitamin E), conjugated linoleic acid (CLA), and minor phospholipids. These molecules play a protective role by scavenging free radicals and interrupting oxidative chain reactions. From a formulation perspective, this is highly significant. Oxidation is one of the primary causes of degradation for many bioactive compounds, particularly polyphenols and unsaturated lipids. The presence of these endogenous antioxidants allows ghee to function as a self-stabilizing system, reducing the need for additional synthetic stabilizers.

This combination of solubilization, interfacial stabilization, molecular association, and intrinsic antioxidant protection makes ghee a uniquely versatile delivery medium. Each class of compound finds its own compatible microenvironment within the lipid matrix—whether dissolved in the core, aligned at the interface, or stabilized within phospholipid domains. Modern pharmaceutical science achieves similar outcomes through carefully engineered systems such as emulsions, liposomes, and self-emulsifying formulations. Yet, in ghee, these principles arise naturally through its composition and behavior during digestion.

What emerges is a picture of remarkable molecular harmony. The lipid matrix of ghee does not merely carry herbal compounds; it actively shapes their stability, release, and absorption. The traditional use of ghee as a carrier for herbal medicines, therefore, reflects a deep empirical understanding—one that aligns closely with the most advanced concepts of contemporary drug delivery science.

6.5. Ghrita as a Proto-Liposomal System

If one were to visualize Ghrita with today's tools—cryo-TEM, DLS, or FTIR—you'd likely detect a spectrum of colloidal structures: microdroplets, vesicles, and lamellar sheets. These are **self-assembled lipid aggregates**, driven by amphiphilic herbal molecules that act as natural surfactants.

The analogy is clear:

Ayurvedic Ghrita	Modern Equivalent	Shared Function
Ghee (triglycerides, phospholipids)	Lipid bilayer / oil core	Solubilization of lipophilic actives
Herbal saponins and glycosides	Natural emulsifiers	Vesicle stabilization
Slow-release upon digestion	Controlled release system	Sustained plasma levels
Deep tissue penetration (Snehana)	Lymphatic absorption / membrane fusion	Targeted delivery

Thus, Ghrita may rightfully be viewed as the **world's earliest lipid vesicular system**—not designed by chemistry, but discovered through intuition and centuries of empirical refinement.

6.6. Ancient China: The Birth of Pill and Powder

In Traditional Chinese Medicine (TCM), healers developed tiny honey pills (蜜丸, mì wán) to preserve herbal extracts, mask unpleasant flavors, and make them portable. They also created powdered medicines for inhalation—an early attempt at delivering drugs directly to the lungs.

Some Chinese remedies were fermented, allowing natural microorganisms to partially "process" plant compounds into more active or less toxic forms before consumption—an early example of bioactivation.

6.7. Egypt, Persia, and the Arab World: The Pharmacy Blossoms

Ancient Egyptians used wine, beer, and milk as carriers for medicines, knowing these liquids could extract and preserve plant actives. They also prepared suppositories—a method still in use today—for local delivery in the rectum or vagina.

During the Islamic Golden Age, Persian and Arab physicians like Avicenna refined the art of syrups, lozenges, and ointments. They also pioneered distillation to extract pure plant oils—a step closer to modern pharmaceutical purity.

6.8. The Slow March to Modern Drug Delivery

For centuries, medicines were crude—plants, minerals, and animal products in basic forms. But the Industrial Revolution and modern chemistry changed everything.

6.8.1. 19th Century: Chemistry Meets Medicine

Scientists learned to isolate pure active ingredients—morphine from opium, quinine from cinchona bark, aspirin from willow bark. These were potent but also dangerous if not dosed carefully. This increased the urgency for controlled delivery.

The first gelatin capsules appeared in the mid-1800s, allowing medicines to be swallowed easily without unpleasant taste. Tablets soon followed—compact, stable, and easy to dose.

6.8.2. Early 20th Century: The Age of Controlled Release

By the early 1900s, pharmacists experimented with coatings to control when a tablet dissolved—for example, making it survive stomach acid and release in the intestine. Ointments, injectable solutions, and inhalers became more refined.

Still, most medicines lacked targeted delivery. Once inside the body, they spread everywhere—good for widespread infections, but bad for diseases where precision mattered, like cancer.

6.9. Why Precision Delivery Matters

Let's imagine you're fighting a fire in one building of a city. You wouldn't spray water across the entire city—you'd focus only on the burning building. Similarly, giving a strong drug to the whole body when only one organ needs it can cause unnecessary "flooding" and damage.

For example:

Cancer chemotherapy can harm healthy cells along with cancer cells.

Steroid medicines can cause severe side effects if distributed everywhere.

Peptide and protein drugs like insulin can be destroyed by stomach acid unless specially protected.

This need for precision—delivering a drug to exactly where it's needed—is what pushed scientists to develop smarter systems.

Chapter

07

Enter the World of Liposomes

Sometimes, great discoveries happen not through grand design, but through simple curiosity—and a touch of serendipity. The story of liposomes begins in the early 1960s at the Babraham Institute in Cambridge, where a British biophysicist named **Dr. Alec D. Bangham** was trying to understand one of biology's most mysterious structures—the **cell membrane**.

Bangham mixed **phospholipids**, the same fat-like molecules that form our cell walls, with water. He wanted to observe how membranes behave, expecting to see a flat film or thin layer. But when he examined the mixture under an **electron microscope**, what appeared stunned him—**tiny, perfectly round bubbles** made of concentric layers, each resembling a miniature version of a biological membrane. These microscopic bubbles enclosed water within them, forming natural compartments.

At first, Bangham and his colleague **R. W. Horne** didn't call them liposomes. In their scientific notes, they used terms such as *"concentric bimolecular lamellae"* or *"multilamellar structures."* Among friends, some even jokingly called them **"Banghasomes"**, after their discoverer. The goal wasn't drug delivery—Bangham was simply building a *model membrane* to study how substances move in and out of cells.

Yet the images he captured were mesmerizing. The layers were so ordered, so cell-like, that other scientists immediately recognized their potential. During one discussion at a Cambridge pub, Bangham's collaborator **Dr. Gerald Weissmann** suggested a name that would soon echo around the scientific world—**"liposome,"** from the Greek *"lipos"* meaning fat and *"soma"* meaning body. The name was catchy, descriptive, and elegant—and it stuck.

What began as an accidental observation soon transformed into one of the most revolutionary ideas in modern medicine. Scientists realized that these microscopic bubbles could **carry drugs** inside them, **protect** them from destruction by stomach acid or enzymes, and **release** them slowly and precisely at the site of action.

Through the 1970s and 1980s, liposomes evolved from scientific curiosities to serious medical tools. Researchers learned to make them smaller, more uniform, and more stable. They discovered ways to attach special molecules to their surfaces, guiding them like guided missiles toward cancer cells or specific tissues.

Then came the clinical breakthrough: in the 1990s, the first liposome-based drug, **Doxil**, was approved for treating cancer. This innovation allowed the powerful chemotherapy drug doxorubicin to reach tumor cells efficiently while minimizing harm to healthy tissue—a milestone that marked the dawn of targeted drug delivery.

Today, liposomes are everywhere—in **vaccines, cosmetics, nutraceuticals, and advanced therapeutics**. They are built from the same materials as our own cells, making them biocompatible, safe, and intelligent. What began as a playful curiosity in a Cambridge lab has become one of the most elegant and impactful technologies in modern science—**tiny bubbles with a big impact**.

This was a turning point in drug delivery history. For the first time, scientists could mimic a living cell's own membrane to transport drugs more safely and effectively.

7.1. The Journey Ahead

From honey-wrapped herbs in ancient Greece to lipid bubbles in modern labs, the goal has always been the same: get the right medicine to the right place at the right time.

In the chapters ahead, we'll explore:

How liposomes are made and work

When the right kind of lipid molecules meet water, something remarkable happens by themselves. Each molecule has a head that loves water and tails that hate it. To keep both sides happy, they arrange in a way where the tails hide from water and the heads stay in contact with it. This forms a delicate two-layered film known as a **lipid bilayer**. When this bilayer bends around and closes upon itself, it creates a tiny sealed sphere—a **liposome**.

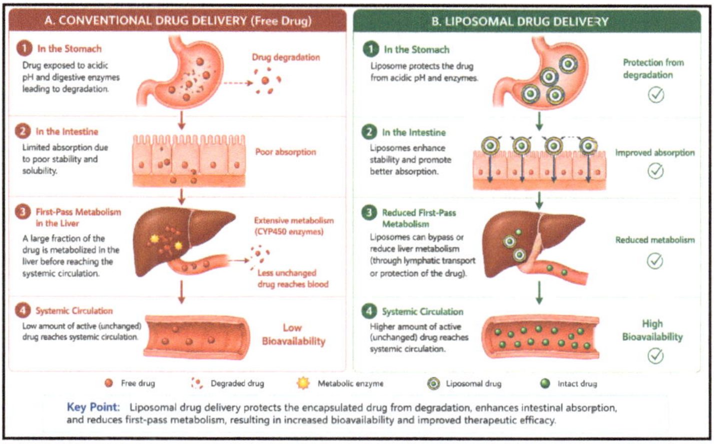

Figure 6. Comparison of conventional and liposomal drug delivery systems.

Schematic illustration comparing conventional drug delivery, where the free drug may undergo degradation in the gastrointestinal tract and extensive first-pass metabolism resulting in reduced bioavailability, with liposomal delivery, where encapsulation within lipid vesicles protects the drug, enhances intestinal absorption, reduces metabolic loss, and improves systemic availability.

Liposomes can be made **with or without cholesterol**, depending on the design and purpose. Cholesterol is often used to tighten and stiffen the membrane, but it is not always necessary. In fact, many modern liposomal systems, especially those meant for nutritional or topical delivery, can achieve exceptional stability and functionality without cholesterol—provided the lipids are carefully chosen and engineered.

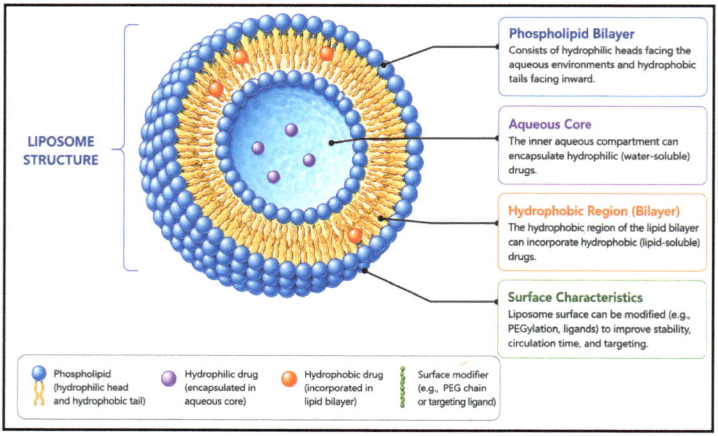

Figure 7. Structure of a liposome.

For me, the preferred starting point is **phosphatidylcholine (PC)** derived from **sunflower**. Sunflower PC forms smooth, flexible, biocompatible bilayers that closely resemble natural cell membranes. It offers an allergen-free, non-GMO alternative to soy PC and can form highly stable vesicles on its own. Other phospholipids can be added to fine-tune texture, charge, or release properties, but the essence of a liposome lies in how these molecules self-assemble in water.

Schematic representation of a liposome composed of a phospholipid bilayer enclosing an aqueous core. Hydrophilic drugs are encapsulated within the inner aqueous compartment, while hydrophobic drugs are incorporated within the lipid bilayer. Surface modifications such as PEGylation or ligand attachment may be used to enhance stability, circulation time, and targeted delivery.

The most classical way to make liposomes—and still one of the most insightful—is the **thin-film hydration method**. Lipids are first dissolved in a clean volatile solvent such as ethanol or chloroform. When the solvent is evaporated, a thin lipid film forms on the wall of the vessel. Adding warm buffer and gently agitating hydrates this film, and as it lifts off, the lipids spontaneously curl into layered vesicles. These multilamellar vesicles are then reduced to a desired size through **extrusion**—passing them through filters with defined pore sizes—until a uniform suspension of nanosized liposomes is achieved.

Over time, newer and more precise techniques have emerged. One of the most important is **microfluidic mixing**, where a stream of lipids dissolved in alcohol meets a stream of water containing the active ingredient inside a narrow microchannel. Within milliseconds, the lipids organize into nanosized vesicles with consistent structure and size distribution. This technique allows exceptional reproducibility and scalability, and it avoids many of the limitations of older batch methods.

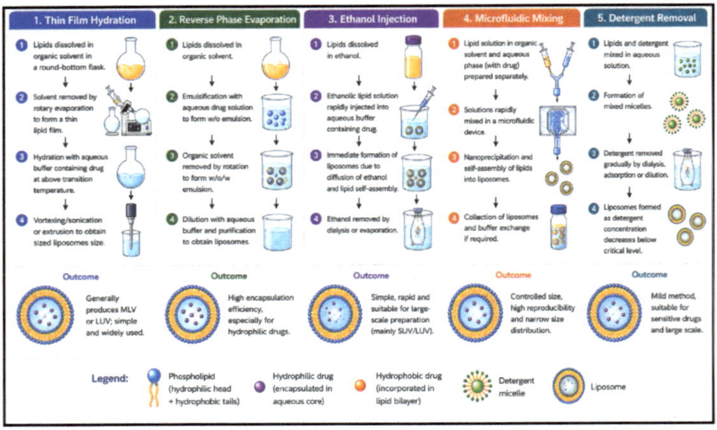

Figure 8. Liposome preparation methods.

Schematic illustration of commonly used techniques for liposome preparation, including thin film hydration, reverse-phase evaporation, ethanol injection, microfluidic mixing, and detergent removal. These methods differ in their mechanisms of vesicle formation, size control, lamellarity, and encapsulation efficiency, enabling the production of liposomes tailored for specific drug delivery applications.

Encapsulating the active ingredient within a liposome depends on its chemical nature. Water-soluble molecules can be trapped in the aqueous interior, while oil-soluble compounds naturally integrate into the bilayer. For certain molecules, especially those that are amphiphilic or pH-sensitive, we can use a process called **remote loading**. In this method, the liposome is first prepared with a controlled internal environment—for example, a pH or ionic gradient—that drives the active compound inside and keeps it there. The result is a high-efficiency loading process with superior retention and controlled release.

Once administered, liposomes behave like microscopic couriers. Their size, surface charge, and composition determine how long they circulate and where they go. Neutral or slightly negative liposomes remain in the bloodstream longer, while those with positive charges interact more with cell membranes. Smaller vesicles, typically around 100 nanometers, travel more efficiently through biological barriers. In cancer and inflammation research, liposomes take advantage of leaky vasculature to accumulate preferentially in diseased tissue—a phenomenon known as the **Enhanced Permeability and Retention (EPR)** effect.

The way a liposome releases its contents can be gradual or precisely triggered. The lipid composition controls the tightness of the bilayer—how easily the active diffuses out. Some systems are designed to respond to specific conditions such as pH, temperature, or enzymes. For example, a pH-responsive liposome can remain stable in the bloodstream but release its contents inside acidic environments like tumors or endosomes. Thermosensitive liposomes open at mild heat, allowing localized delivery, and enzyme-responsive liposomes release their payload where specific enzymes are abundant, such as in inflamed tissues or wounds.

In formulation research, each batch of liposomes is carefully characterized. Their size and uniformity are measured using **dynamic light scattering (DLS)**, surface charge is determined through **zeta potential**, and their internal structure is visualized using **cryo-electron microscopy**. The encapsulation efficiency and leakage rate are quantified over time to confirm stability. When a dry, portable form is needed, liposomes are gently **freeze-dried** with protective sugars like trehalose or sucrose, which create a glassy matrix that preserves the bilayer and allows the liposome to revive fully when rehydrated.

A major challenge for decades was how to make liposomes that remain stable in solid form—not as delicate suspensions. Through persistent work, my team developed **Metazome® technology**, a next-generation liposomal platform that produces **true, solid-state liposomes** capable of withstanding drying, storage, and even compression into beadlets or tablets. Built primarily on sunflower phosphatidylcholine and stabilized through unique molecular architecture rather than cholesterol, Metazome® liposomes retain their bilayer integrity and instantly rehydrate to functional vesicles when dispersed in water. This approach opened a new dimension for liposomal nutraceuticals and pharmaceuticals—systems that combine biological intelligence with industrial stability.

Liposomes succeed because they mimic nature's design while extending human control over it. They **protect** delicate molecules from degradation, **navigate** intelligently through the body, and **release** their actives exactly when and where they are needed. Whether they exist as a fluid nanosuspension or as a dry, rehydratable Metazome® liposomes represent a perfect marriage of chemistry, physics, and biology—tiny self-assembling bubbles that continue to reshape modern medicine and nutrition.

7.2. What Happens When a Liposome Enters the Body

The story of a liposome doesn't end when it is created in the lab—in fact, that's where its real journey begins. Imagine releasing millions of tiny, intelligent couriers into the human body, each carrying a precious cargo and a mission: to deliver it safely, intact, and precisely where it's needed.

When a liposomal formulation is swallowed, injected, or applied on the skin, the first thing it encounters is the complex environment of the body—full of enzymes, pH changes, biological barriers, and immune defenses. Each of these conditions tries to interfere with the liposome's mission, yet a well-designed vesicle knows how to navigate them.

If taken **orally**, liposomes face one of the harshest environments—the stomach. The acidic pH and digestive enzymes can easily destroy most molecules, but liposomes built from natural phospholipids form a protective barrier that resists degradation long enough to reach the intestine. Once in the small intestine, bile salts and phospholipases start interacting with the liposomes. Some break open and release the encapsulated actives, which can then diffuse across the intestinal wall. Others merge with the lipid membranes of intestinal cells or with micelles, allowing the cargo to enter through passive diffusion or endocytosis. Because the lipids in the liposome resemble those in the intestinal lining, they are recognized as "self"—not as foreign invaders—and this similarity greatly improves the absorption of otherwise poorly bioavailable compounds.

When liposomes are delivered **intravenously**, their story is slightly different but equally fascinating. As soon as they enter the bloodstream, plasma proteins rush toward them, forming what scientists call a **protein corona**. This coating can either be beneficial or problematic, depending on how the liposome is designed. Non-PEGylated or highly charged liposomes are quickly recognized and engulfed by the macrophages of the **reticuloendothelial system (RES)**—mainly in the liver, spleen, and bone marrow. This is why early liposomal drugs disappeared from the bloodstream within minutes. Over the years, researchers learned how to modify the surface, reducing the charge and adding a thin layer of hydrophilic polymers such as PEG to create what are known as **stealth liposomes**. These stealthy vesicles avoid immune detection and can circulate for hours or even days, distributing widely before being cleared.

Inside the body, the journey of each liposome depends on its **size, charge, and composition**. Smaller liposomes (around 100 nanometers) can slip through the tiniest gaps in the blood vessel walls, especially in tissues that have leaky vasculature such as tumors, inflamed regions, or liver sinusoids. This natural phenomenon is called the **Enhanced Permeability and Retention (EPR) effect**, and it's one of the key reasons liposomal drug delivery became so successful in oncology.

Once a liposome reaches its destination tissue, the next step is **cellular entry**. Cells can internalize liposomes through several mechanisms, but the most common is **endocytosis**—the cell membrane gently folds around the liposome, swallowing it into an internal compartment known as an **endosome**. Inside this tiny vesicle, the environment gradually becomes more acidic. For liposomes designed with **pH-sensitive phospholipids**, this change in acidity triggers the bilayer to destabilize or fuse with the endosomal membrane, releasing the drug directly into the cytoplasm. Other liposomes simply degrade slowly, leaking the active compound in a controlled fashion, allowing the cell to take it up gradually.

In some cases, the liposomes don't enter the cell at all but **fuse directly with the cell membrane**, much like two soap bubbles merging into one. When this happens, the drug moves straight into the cell's interior, bypassing the usual uptake pathways. This mechanism is particularly useful for lipophilic compounds and antioxidants that need to act within the lipid regions of membranes or mitochondria.

After completing their task, liposomes—being made of natural materials such as phosphatidylcholine—are metabolized just like dietary fats. Enzymes break them down into fatty acids, glycerol, and choline, all of which are either reused by the body or safely eliminated. This biodegradability is one of the most beautiful aspects of liposomes: they do their job, and then they simply disappear without leaving behind any toxic residues.

In topical or cosmetic applications, liposomes interact with the **stratum corneum**, the outermost layer of the skin. Here, their behavior is guided by size and flexibility. Smaller and more deformable liposomes can penetrate deeper into the epidermis, while larger ones remain near the surface, forming a reservoir that slowly releases the active ingredient. This dual action—surface protection and deep delivery—explains why liposomal systems have become a foundation in advanced skincare.

The pharmacokinetic life of a liposome can be summarized in three words—**protect, navigate, and release**. First, the liposome protects its cargo from degradation. Second, it navigates intelligently through biological barriers, sometimes sneaking through natural gaps, sometimes merging with cell membranes. Finally, it releases the active compound exactly where it is needed—not too early, not too late.

What happens next depends on the formulation goal. In medicine, the focus is on precision and therapeutic effect. In nutrition, it is on enhanced absorption and stability. In cosmetics, it is on controlled penetration and hydration. But in every case, the underlying principle is the same—the liposome becomes an elegant messenger, designed to cross boundaries that free molecules never could.

That is why liposomes are more than just carriers; they are **communicators between chemistry and biology**. Each one is a self-assembled world—built from natural phospholipids, powered by molecular organization, and guided by physics—yet their impact unfolds at the level of life itself.

The different types of liposomal systems

7.3 The Different Faces of Liposomes

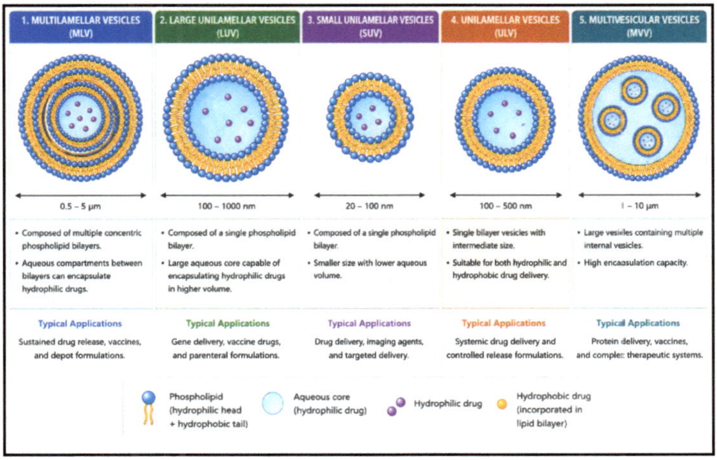

Figure 9. Types of liposomes based on size and lamellarity.

When we speak of liposomes, we often imagine a single type of bubble, but in truth there are many variations—each designed with a specific purpose in mind. Just as the same basic element carbon can form graphite, diamond, or graphene depending on how its atoms are arranged, liposomes reveal completely different personalities depending on how their molecules assemble and how scientists choose to modify them.

Schematic representation of different classes of liposomes, including multilamellar vesicles (MLV), large unilamellar vesicles (LUV), small unilamellar vesicles (SUV), unilamellar vesicles (ULV), and multivesicular vesicles (MVV). These liposomes differ in the number of phospholipid bilayers, size, and internal structure, which influence their drug encapsulation capacity and suitability for various drug delivery applications.

7.4. Multilamellar and Unilamellar Liposomes – The Foundation

The earliest liposomes observed by Alec Bangham were **multilamellar vesicles (MLVs)**. Under the microscope, they looked like onions—multiple lipid bilayers wrapped concentrically around a watery core. Each layer could hold lipophilic compounds between its membranes and hydrophilic molecules within the water compartments. These MLVs are mechanically robust and easy to prepare but relatively large, often several hundred nanometers or even micrometers in diameter. Because of their size, they are not ideal for intravenous or deep-tissue applications, yet they remain useful when a slow release or topical action is desired.

To achieve more controlled behavior, researchers developed **unilamellar vesicles (ULVs)**, which contain only one bilayer surrounding a single aqueous core.

These can be either **large unilamellar vesicles (LUVs)**, typically 100–1000 nm, or **small unilamellar vesicles (SUVs)**, usually 30–100 nm. SUVs are particularly interesting because their small size allows them to penetrate biological barriers and circulate longer in the bloodstream. They are the workhorses of most medical and nutraceutical applications today.

7.5. Stealth Liposomes – The Art of Disguise

When the first liposomal drugs were injected into patients, researchers discovered a problem: the body's immune system cleared them almost instantly. Macrophages in the liver and spleen recognized the vesicles as foreign particles. The solution came in the form of **surface camouflage**. By attaching flexible, water-loving chains of polyethylene glycol (PEG) to the surface, scientists created what are now known as **stealth liposomes**. PEG forms a soft protective cloud that prevents proteins from binding to the surface and tagging the liposome for removal. These stealth liposomes can circulate for many hours, giving the drug far more time to reach its target tissues.

PEGylation, however, is not the only way to achieve stealth. In recent years, alternative natural coatings such as oligosaccharides, zwitterionic lipids, and even biomimetic membranes have been explored to create long-circulating systems that are better tolerated in sensitive patients.

7.6. Targeted Liposomes – Precision Delivery

While stealth extends circulation, **targeted liposomes** add direction. These are vesicles equipped with molecules on their surface that act as address labels. The label can be an antibody, a small peptide, a vitamin such as folate, or a sugar that binds to a specific receptor on a target cell. When the liposome encounters the correct cell, the ligand–receptor interaction triggers attachment and often internalization by endocytosis. In cancer therapy, for example, this strategy allows drugs to concentrate in tumor cells while sparing healthy tissue. In cosmetic and nutraceutical systems, targeting peptides or plant-derived ligands can be used to enhance uptake into skin or intestinal epithelial cells, improving bioavailability without toxicity.

7.7. Stimuli-Responsive Liposomes – Intelligent Release

Some liposomes are designed to act only under certain conditions. These **stimuli-responsive** systems are the intelligent generation of delivery vehicles.

- **pH-sensitive liposomes** remain stable in the bloodstream but destabilize in acidic environments such as tumors or intracellular endosomes, releasing the active at exactly the right moment. (pH-sensitive liposomes do not respond to "any" acidic environment—they are engineered to respond within a very specific and narrow pH window. This distinction explains how they can remain stable in the stomach yet become active in biological compartments such as tumors or endosomes. The gastric environment is extremely acidic, typically around pH 1–3, whereas the environments that trigger pH-responsive liposomes are only mildly acidic, generally in the range of pH 5.0–6.5. Lipids used in these systems are carefully selected so that their protonation—and the resulting membrane destabilization—occurs only within this mild acidity range. As a result, the bilayer can remain intact in the highly acidic stomach but undergo structural changes when it encounters the subtler pH conditions inside cells or diseased tissues. For oral delivery, additional design elements reinforce this stability. The lipid composition is optimized to create a tightly packed, less permeable membrane that resists rapid disruption. Surface-associated components or protective matrices can further shield the vesicle from direct acid exposure. Moreover, gastric transit is relatively short, allowing kinetically stable liposomes to pass through before significant degradation occurs. It is also important to recognize that bile salts in the intestine are often more disruptive to lipid structures than gastric acid itself. Well-designed systems therefore balance resistance to gastric conditions with the ability to reorganize or interact effectively in the intestinal environment, where absorption takes place. In this way, pH-responsive liposomes are not broadly acid-sensitive but precisely tuned systems—stable in harsh gastric conditions, yet capable of responding to the specific, milder acidity that defines their intended site of action.)

- **Thermo-sensitive liposomes** use phospholipids whose bilayers become fluid at mild fever-like temperatures (around 40 °C). Local heating of a tumor can trigger a rapid, localized drug burst.
- **Enzyme-responsive liposomes** exploit the presence of phospholipases or proteases in inflamed or infected tissues to break down their membranes.
- **Redox-responsive systems** contain disulfide linkages that open in the high-glutathione environment inside cells, ensuring cytosolic delivery.

These systems transform liposomes from passive carriers into smart devices that sense their surroundings.

7.8. Cationic and Ionizable Liposomes – Gene and RNA Delivery

Another specialized category is the **cationic or ionizable liposome**, used primarily for delivering nucleic acids such as DNA, siRNA, or mRNA. These vesicles have positively charged surfaces that bind the negatively charged genetic material, forming compact structures that can fuse with cell membranes. Ionizable lipids, in particular, remain neutral in blood (reducing toxicity) but become positively charged in the acidic environment of endosomes, helping the nucleic acid escape into the cytoplasm. This principle forms the foundation of modern **lipid nanoparticle (LNP)** vaccines and therapeutics—a close cousin of the classical liposome, but with a non-lamellar inner core.

7.9. Deformable and Elastic Liposomes – Crossing Barriers

For skin and mucosal delivery, **elastic or deformable liposomes**—sometimes called *transferosomes* or *niosomes* (when built from non-ionic surfactants instead of phospholipids)—bring a unique advantage. Their bilayers contain flexible edge activators that let them squeeze through microscopic pores much smaller than their own diameter. This ability allows deep penetration through the stratum corneum and mucosal surfaces, carrying both hydrophilic and lipophilic actives efficiently.

7.10. Solid-State and Beadlet Liposomes – The Next Leap

One of the most significant challenges in liposome technology has always been physical stability. Traditional liposomes exist as aqueous dispersions that are sensitive to temperature, oxidation, and microbial growth. The need for refrigeration and short shelf life made them impractical for many applications outside hospitals.

To overcome this, the field moved toward **solid-state liposomes**, where the vesicle architecture is preserved even in a dry form. The process requires precise control of lipid composition, water removal, and protective excipients to prevent bilayer collapse. My work on **Metazome® technology** was developed to address exactly this problem. Instead of depending on cholesterol for rigidity, Metazome® systems rely on molecular engineering of sunflower-derived phosphatidylcholine and other natural stabilizers to create a *compressible yet rehydratable bilayer matrix.* In this architecture, each liposome is embedded in a supportive micro-environment that holds its shape during drying and tableting. Upon contact with water, the bilayer instantly reconstructs, restoring a true nanoscale liposome with its encapsulated active still intact.

This innovation bridges the gap between biological sophistication and industrial practicality—making it possible to formulate **liposomal powders, beadlets, and chewable solids** that maintain the same functional integrity as liquid suspensions. In nutraceuticals and functional foods, this opens doors to entirely new dosage forms that were once impossible with fragile wet liposomes.

7.11. Hybrid and Multifunctional Systems – The Frontier

The modern face of liposomal science is increasingly hybrid. Researchers now integrate liposomes with **polymers**, **metallic nanostructures**, or **biopolymers** to achieve multiple functions: sustained release, imaging contrast, or synergistic delivery. Some systems combine

liposomes with solid-lipid nanoparticles, creating core–shell architectures that merge the advantages of both. Others include **magnetically responsive nanoparticles** or **quantum dots** within the bilayer for theranostic applications, uniting therapy and diagnostics in a single system.

Each of these liposomal forms—from the simple onion-like multilamellar vesicle to the dry, intelligent Metazome® beadlet—represents a chapter in the ongoing evolution of drug delivery science. The versatility of the lipid bilayer allows us to engineer function at every scale: stability, targeting, responsiveness, and compatibility.

The real beauty of liposomes lies in their simplicity: a natural membrane reborn as a technological masterpiece. Whether it circulates silently in blood, penetrates deep into tissue, or rests on a shelf as a stable powder waiting to come alive again, the liposome remains one of the most elegant inventions in modern chemistry—a small bubble that continues to make an ever-growing impact.

Chapter

08

How Liposomes Differ from Other Delivery Systems

When we talk about "drug delivery systems," many people imagine all of them as tiny capsules doing the same job. But in reality, each system is like a different type of vehicle—all designed to carry passengers, but suited to different roads and destinations.

Liposomes are one such vehicle—elegant and intelligent—but they share the road with others like micelles, niosomes, phytosomes, solid lipid nanoparticles, and polymeric carriers. To really appreciate what makes liposomes special, it helps to compare them with these fellow travelers.

8.1. Liposomes – The Miniature Cells

Think of liposomes as tiny **artificial cells**, made mostly from the same materials our own cell membranes are built from—phospholipids. When these molecules meet water, they form a thin membrane that curls into a sphere. Inside is water, outside is water, and the membrane itself can hold oily or fat-loving substances.

That makes liposomes unique—they can carry **both** water-soluble and fat-soluble nutrients or medicines at the same time. For example, vitamin C (which dissolves in water) and curcumin (which dissolves in oil) can both be carried together in the same liposomal structure.

They are also biodegradable and biocompatible—the body recognizes them as natural and eventually breaks them down just like it would digest healthy fats. Because of this, liposomes are widely used not only in medicine but also in nutrition and cosmetics.

You could say that liposomes are like **electric cars** in the vehicle analogy—clean, efficient, and designed with nature's principles in mind.

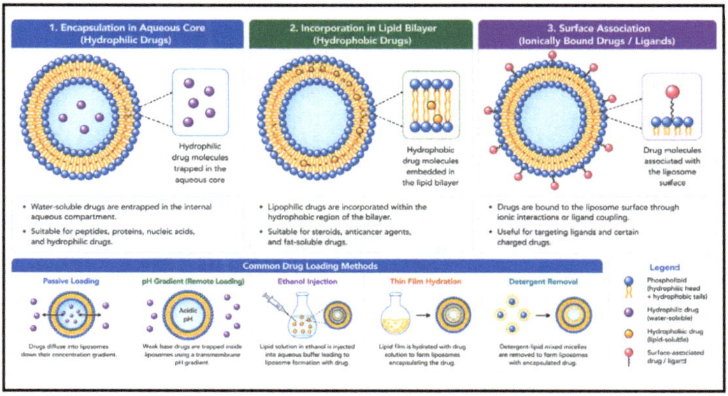

Figure 10. Drug encapsulation and loading in liposomes.

Schematic illustration of the different modes of drug incorporation into liposomes, including encapsulation of hydrophilic drugs within the aqueous core, incorporation of hydrophobic drugs within the lipid bilayer, and surface association of drugs or ligands. Common loading approaches are also depicted, highlighting strategies used to achieve efficient drug delivery based on physicochemical properties.

8.2. Micelles – The Soap Bubbles of Chemistry

Before liposomes, chemists worked with something simpler called **micelles.** A micelle is what happens when soap or detergent molecules meet water. The oily parts of the molecules hide inside, and the water-loving parts stay on the outside. This structure can trap oily dirt or fat-soluble drugs in its core and carry them through water.

Micelles are wonderful for dissolving and transporting oil-based compounds like vitamin E or coenzyme Q10, but they have one weakness—they don't have a water-filled center, so they cannot carry water-soluble compounds. Also, micelles fall apart when diluted too much, which can happen inside the body.

If liposomes are like a **sealed courier truck**, micelles are more like **open pickup vans**—perfect for carrying oily cargo, but not for fragile, water-based materials.

8.3. Niosomes – The Synthetic Cousins

Niosomes look and behave very much like liposomes but are made from **non-ionic surfactants** instead of natural phospholipids. They are like a **sturdier, more synthetic**

version of liposomes—good for skin applications and often cheaper to make.

For example, in skincare, niosomes are used to deliver actives like peptides or botanical extracts through the skin barrier. They are flexible and can squeeze through pores that are smaller than themselves. However, because their materials are more synthetic, they are not as naturally accepted by the body as phospholipid-based liposomes, especially for injectable or internal use.

Imagine niosomes as **plastic boats**—strong, reliable, and inexpensive—while liposomes are **organic wooden boats**, shaped by nature and more compatible with living systems.

8.4. Phytosomes – Plant Molecules with a Passport

Phytosomes are a very different concept. They are not hollow bubbles like liposomes. Instead, they are **complexes formed between plant molecules and phospholipids**.

Take curcumin from turmeric or quercetin from onions—both have poor absorption when taken on their own. In a phytosome, each plant molecule forms a chemical handshake with a phospholipid, making it more soluble and better absorbed in the intestine.

Phytosomes don't "encapsulate" the molecule; they bond with it. Think of it like getting a passport that allows the plant molecule to cross the biological border easily. A curcumin molecule in a phytosome is no longer traveling alone—it's riding piggyback on a lipid partner that knows the route.

So, if liposomes are **delivery trucks**, phytosomes are **VIP travel passes** that help plant compounds pass customs faster.

8.5. Solid Lipid Nanoparticles – The Ice Cubes of the Nano World

Solid lipid nanoparticles, or SLNs, are another way to deliver drugs or nutrients, especially oily ones. Instead of being a hollow sphere like a liposome, an SLN is a **solid fat particle** at body temperature, with a drug trapped inside.

When taken orally or applied on the skin, the solid fat slowly melts or erodes, releasing the active compound over time. This makes SLNs great for sustained release—a bit like an **ice cube that slowly melts**, releasing flavor into your drink over time.

However, since they're made of solid fat, they're not suitable for water-soluble drugs, and their internal structure is much less flexible than a liposome's bilayer. They're more like frozen capsules than dynamic membranes.

8.6. Polymeric Nanoparticles – The Slow-Release Capsules

Polymeric nanoparticles are made from biodegradable polymers such as PLGA. When drugs are embedded in these tiny spheres, they are slowly released as the polymer breaks down. This technology is widely used for injections that need to work for weeks or months—for example, in some hormone therapies or long-acting painkillers.

They act like **slow-dissolving candies**—once swallowed or injected, they melt gradually, releasing the drug bit by bit. They're ideal for long-term, steady release, but not for delicate or natural molecules that can't handle the harsh polymerization process.

In contrast, liposomes handle fragile, water-sensitive, or bioactive molecules much more gently, mimicking biological conditions.

8.7. Lipid Nanoparticles (LNPs) – The Genetic Messengers

During the COVID-19 vaccine era, many people heard the term **LNPs**, or **lipid nanoparticles**. Though often confused with liposomes, they are not quite the same. LNPs are built to deliver genetic material like mRNA, not small molecules or nutrients.

They don't have a hollow water core like liposomes; instead, they contain a **dense, complexed interior** where the RNA is tightly packed with special ionizable lipids. These lipids stay neutral in the bloodstream but become positively charged inside cells, helping the mRNA escape into the cytoplasm.

Think of an LNP as a **smart rocket capsule** that carries delicate instructions (like mRNA) into the cell, releases them, and then vanishes. Liposomes, in contrast, are **multi-purpose couriers**—they can carry almost anything: vitamins, plant extracts, or pharmaceutical drugs.

8.8. Nanoemulsions – The Salad Dressings of Drug Delivery

A **nanoemulsion** is nothing more than a very fine oil-in-water or water-in-oil mixture stabilized by surfactants. In a way, it's just a highly refined **salad dressing** where oil droplets are so tiny they remain suspended for months without separating.

Nanoemulsions are great for increasing the bioavailability of fat-soluble vitamins and plant oils. They're simple to make, taste pleasant, and can be used in beverages or creams. But because they don't have a bilayer structure, they cannot protect or slowly release drugs the way liposomes do.

A nanoemulsion delivers quickly—like an **energy drink** that hits fast—whereas a liposome is more like a **time-release capsule**, delivering steadily and precisely.

8.9. Cubosomes and Hexosomes – The Honeycombs of Nanoworld

Cubosomes and hexosomes are fascinating structures with **three-dimensional internal networks** of lipid and water channels—they look like microscopic honeycombs. Because of their large internal surface area, they can hold a lot of material and release it slowly as the channels break down.

They are being explored for advanced skin delivery, inhalation therapy, and even food encapsulation. But they are difficult to make consistently, and their thick, gel-like texture limits where they can be used. Think of them as **complex honeycombs** rather than simple bubbles—powerful but not always easy to control.

8.10. So, What Makes Liposomes Stand Out?

After comparing all these systems, the difference becomes clear. Liposomes are the **most balanced and biomimetic** of all—they behave like living membranes, interact gracefully with cells, and can carry both water- and fat-soluble materials.

They can be made from **natural sunflower phosphatidylcholine**, without the need for cholesterol, and can now even exist as **solid powders or beadlets** that rehydrate instantly—as in **Metazome® technology**—giving them long shelf life and industrial stability without losing their biological intelligence.

If micelles are soap bubbles, nanoemulsions are salad dressings, and polymeric nanoparticles are time-release capsules, then liposomes are the **Swiss Army knife** of drug delivery—natural, adaptable, intelligent, and now, thanks to modern science, more practical than ever before.

That's why, even after sixty years of research and countless competing technologies, liposomes continue to hold their place at the heart of modern delivery science—small bubbles with a big, ever-growing impact.

8.11. The Phase Transition Temperature (T_m) – When a Membrane Comes Alive

If you could zoom in close enough to watch the surface of a liposome, you'd see something remarkable—a landscape that changes its personality with temperature. At one temperature it behaves like a stiff waxy shell, and at another, it turns into a flowing, flexible film. That change point is known as the **phase transition temperature**, or $\mathbf{T_m}$.

Just like ice melts to water at 0 °C, the lipids in a membrane undergo their own molecular "melting." Below T_m, the hydrocarbon tails of the phospholipids are tightly packed and ordered, forming what's called the **gel phase** (also called *solid-ordered phase*, symbolized L_β). Above T_m, thermal energy loosens the bonds and the tails begin to rotate and flex freely, transforming the bilayer into the **liquid-crystalline phase** (*liquid-disordered phase*, L_α).

At this moment, the membrane becomes alive—flexible, dynamic, and permeable.

The beauty is that this is not a single number for all liposomes; it depends entirely on the lipid composition.

8.11.1. What Exactly Happens at T_m

Each phospholipid molecule has two tails made of fatty acids. When the temperature is low, these tails are straight and neatly aligned, like pencils in a box. As the temperature rises, the tails start to bend (due to cis double bonds in unsaturated fatty acids) and jiggle more.

At a certain point, the thermal energy is enough to disrupt the ordered packing—the tails start "melting" and moving freely. The distance between lipid molecules increases by 10–20%, and the membrane thickness decreases slightly. This structural rearrangement is the **gel-to-liquid crystalline transition**—the moment the bilayer breathes freely.

This transition is sharp and detectable. If you use **Differential Scanning Calorimetry (DSC)**—a technique that measures how much heat a sample absorbs as it's warmed—you can see a sharp peak at T_m. That peak is the membrane's equivalent of a heartbeat—a direct measurement of its molecular mobility.

For example:

- **Dipalmitylphosphatidylcholine (DPPC)**, a saturated phospholipid, has a T_m around **41 °C**.
- **Dioleoylphosphatidylcholine (DOPC)**, which contains unsaturated tails, has a T_m around **–20 °C**—it's already fluid at room temperature.

- **Hydrogenated soy PC** or **egg PC** can have T_m values anywhere between **–5 °C and 55 °C**, depending on the degree of saturation and chain length.

Thus, by choosing different lipid types, you can *tune* the membrane's transition temperature—and therefore its fluidity and permeability—just as a musician tunes an instrument.

8.11.2. Why T_m Matters in Liposomes

The phase transition temperature defines almost everything about how a liposome behaves—from how tightly it holds its cargo to how easily it merges with cells.

a. Drug Release and Retention

Below T_m (in the gel phase), lipids are tightly packed, forming a rigid barrier. Leakage of water-soluble drugs is minimal. That's why liposomes designed for **slow, sustained release** are often made with high-T_m lipids.

Above T_m (liquid phase), the membrane becomes more fluid and permeable, and drugs diffuse out faster. This property is used intentionally in **thermo-sensitive liposomes**—formulations that remain sealed in the bloodstream but open up when a mild heat (around 42 °C) is applied to a tumor or target tissue. The elevated temperature locally crosses T_m, increasing permeability and releasing the drug precisely where needed.

For instance, *ThermoDox®* (a clinical liposomal doxorubicin) uses DPPC and lysolipids with a transition temperature tuned around **40–42 °C**, so it releases the drug under mild hyperthermia while staying stable at body temperature (37 °C). This is a perfect example of T_m used as a biological switch.

b. Fusion and Cellular Uptake

Membranes that are near their T_m are more fusogenic—they can merge more easily with other membranes. That's because at T_m, the bilayer is in a "softened" state with mixed gel and liquid regions, creating defects where fusion can start. Liposomes designed to deliver materials inside cells often exploit this property: choosing a lipid composition with a T_m slightly below body temperature ensures the membrane remains flexible enough to interact with cellular surfaces without collapsing.

c. Stability During Storage

T_m also governs shelf stability. Liposomes stored below their transition temperature are more rigid and less prone to oxidation or aggregation. However, if the storage temperature fluctuates around T_m, small variations can repeatedly expand and contract the membrane, leading to leakage. For this reason, industrial formulations often select lipids whose T_m is **10 °C higher than room temperature** or much lower, depending on the desired consistency (liquid or solid).

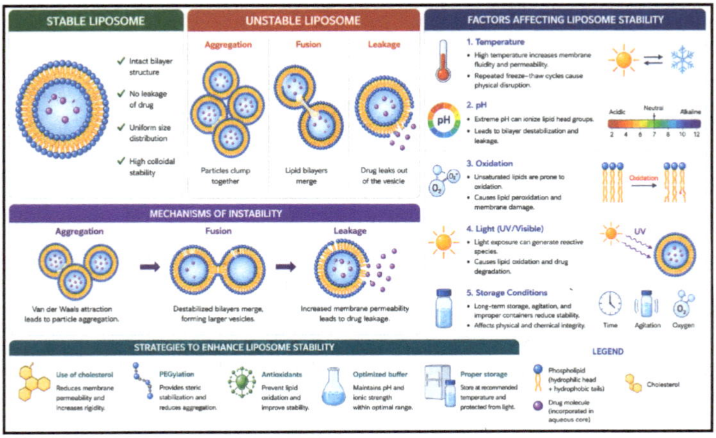

Figure 11. Factors affecting liposome stability.

Schematic illustration of the physical, chemical, and environmental factors influencing liposome stability, including temperature, pH, oxidation, light exposure, and storage conditions. Instability may result in aggregation, fusion, or leakage of encapsulated drug, while appropriate formulation strategies such as cholesterol incorporation, PEGylation, and optimized storage conditions can enhance liposome stability and shelf-life.

8.11.3. Controlling T_m: The Lipid Designer's Toolkit

Scientists can manipulate T_m like an artist playing with color. Here are the key levers:

- **Fatty Acid Chain Length:** Longer chains mean stronger van der Waals forces and higher T_m. (E.g., DMPC → 23 °C; DPPC → 41 °C; DSPC → 55 °C.)

- **Degree of Unsaturation:** Each double bond introduces a kink, preventing tight packing and lowering T_m dramatically.
- **Head Group Composition:** Phosphatidylethanolamine (PE) forms more compact bilayers (higher T_m) than phosphatidylcholine (PC), which is more fluid.
- **Inclusion of Cholesterol:** Cholesterol flattens the transition curve, broadening it and eliminating the sharp melting point. It orders the fluid phase and disorders the gel phase, making the membrane more uniformly fluid across temperatures. (In your sunflower-PC systems that exclude cholesterol, T_m remains sharp and well-defined.)
- **Hydration and pH:** More water and neutral pH promote fluidity; dehydration or ionic changes can shift T_m upward.

By combining these variables, one can fine-tune the T_m of a liposomal system to match a desired application—from **stable room-temperature nutraceutical powders** to **heat-triggered drug carriers**.

8.11.4. Visualizing the Transition—A Molecular "Dance"

Imagine a crowd of people standing shoulder-to-shoulder on a cold morning (the gel phase). As the sun rises and warms them, everyone starts to loosen their stance, sway, and move their arms (the liquid-crystalline phase). The crowd expands slightly, and there's more room for motion—but the group still holds together. That's what happens at T_m.

Physically, you can see it as:

- **Volume increase** of the bilayer by ~4%.
- **Thickness decrease** by ~1 nm.
- **Area per lipid molecule** increasing from ~45 Å² to ~65 Å².

These subtle molecular changes collectively transform the entire liposome's flexibility, permeability, and shape.

In a laboratory, if you warm a liposomal suspension slowly through its T_m, you'll often see the solution turn slightly less opaque—light scattering decreases as vesicles become more uniform. Under the microscope, liposomes become more spherical and fluid, occasionally forming transient "ripple phases"—small waves across their surface that shimmer like the ripples on a lake warmed by morning light.

Chapter 09

The Story of the First FDA-Approved Liposomal Drug

9.1. From Curiosity to Cure

In the 1960s, Alec Bangham and R. W. Horne looked through an electron microscope at thin films of lecithin and saw something astonishing—perfectly round, layered bubbles of fat enclosing water. They called them *"multilamellar smectic mesophases."*

Later, when a visiting biophysicist joked that they looked like tiny "liposomes," the name stuck.

At that time, nobody imagined that these fragile little vesicles would one day change the landscape of modern chemotherapy. The discovery was considered a biochemical curiosity—elegant but impractical. Yet within three decades, these same bubbles would give birth to the **first FDA-approved liposomal drug**: *Doxil*®.

9.2. A Dangerous Molecule in Search of a Safe Journey

The active ingredient behind this revolution was **doxorubicin**, a powerful anthracycline antibiotic discovered in the 1960s from *Streptomyces peucetius*. It was a medical marvel—it could stop cancer cells from dividing by intercalating into DNA—but it was also devastatingly toxic to the heart.

Physicians faced a cruel dilemma: the drug that could save a life could also silently damage the patient's heart muscle with each dose.

Scientists began asking a new kind of question—not *"What drug should we give?"* but *"How should we give it?"*

And this question led them to liposomes.

9.3. The Liposome Renaissance of the 1980s

Through the 1970s and 1980s, researchers like **Demetrios Papahadjopoulos** at UCSF and **Alain Thierry** in France worked to make liposomes more stable and clinically viable. They discovered that if you made the liposomes with **phosphatidylcholine and cholesterol**, the membranes became tighter and less leaky.

But another barrier soon emerged—literally. Once injected, liposomes were quickly recognized by the immune system's **reticuloendothelial system (RES)**—mainly the liver and spleen—and cleared within minutes. The body's cleanup cells treated them like debris, not medicine.

The solution would come from a simple but revolutionary addition: a stealth coating.

9.4. Stealth Liposomes – Hiding in Plain Sight

In the late 1980s, scientists at **Hadassah Medical Center (Jerusalem)** and **Liposome Technology Inc. (Menlo Park, California)** developed a way to cloak liposomes with a polymer called **polyethylene glycol (PEG)**.

This "PEGylation" created a slippery, hydrophilic shield around the liposome, preventing blood proteins from binding and immune cells from recognizing them.

These **"stealth liposomes"** could circulate for many hours, even days—a record compared to the few minutes of earlier systems. That longer circulation meant more of the encapsulated drug would reach tumors through their leaky, fragile blood vessels—a phenomenon known as the **enhanced permeability and retention (EPR) effect**.

Inside these stealth liposomes, the team loaded **doxorubicin hydrochloride** using a clever *remote loading* technique. By establishing a **transmembrane ammonium sulfate gradient**, they could actively drive doxorubicin molecules into the liposome interior, forming stable drug–sulfate complexes.

Encapsulation efficiency exceeded 95%, and leakage was minimal even during storage.

The new formulation was christened **Doxil®** in the United States and **Caelyx®** in Europe.

9.5. The Birth of Doxil – A Triumph of Delivery Science

In 1995, after rigorous testing, **the U.S. Food and Drug Administration (FDA) approved Doxil**, making it the **first liposomal drug in history** to reach the market.

It was a triumph of formulation over molecular reinvention—the same doxorubicin molecule, but now delivered safely and intelligently.

Doxil's **pharmacokinetics were unlike anything seen before**:

- Circulation half-life extended from minutes to **over 50 hours**.
- The drug selectively accumulated in tumor tissues while sparing healthy ones.
- Most remarkably, **cardiotoxicity plummeted**—patients could receive effective doses without heart failure.

Clinically, Doxil was first approved for **AIDS-related Kaposi's sarcoma**, later for **ovarian and breast cancer**, and eventually for **multiple myeloma** (in combination with bortezomib).

The liposome had turned a toxic drug into a manageable therapy—an idea that soon reshaped pharmaceutical research worldwide.

9.6. How Doxil Works – A Journey Through the Body

When injected, Doxil particles (around **100 nm in diameter**) circulate in plasma as long-lived stealth vesicles.

They slowly leak doxorubicin inside the tumor microenvironment, where the **leaky vasculature and poor lymphatic drainage** trap the liposomes (EPR effect).

As tumor cells engulf the vesicles or experience drug diffusion from their surface, doxorubicin is released locally, damaging tumor DNA while sparing most normal tissue.

In essence, the liposome acts like a **molecular courier with a time lock**—carrying a dangerous payload safely until it reaches its destination.

9.7. A Turning Point in Pharmaceutical Thinking

Doxil did more than help cancer patients; it **changed the mindset of drug development**.

For the first time, pharmaceutical success wasn't about discovering a new chemical entity—it was about **engineering the journey** of an old one.

The FDA approval validated the field of nanomedicine. Dozens of liposomal and nanoparticle-based drugs soon followed:

- **Ambisome® (liposomal amphotericin B)** for fungal infections

- **DepoCyt® (liposomal cytarabine)** for meningitis
- **Onivyde® (liposomal irinotecan)** for pancreatic cancer
- and many others.

Each of these owes its lineage to Doxil—the pioneer that proved that a **nanoscopic shell of fat** could transform the meaning of a drug.

9.8. Legacy and Lessons

The story of Doxil is not just about cancer therapy; it's about a **shift in philosophy**—from fighting disease to understanding delivery.

It showed that how a molecule travels determines how it heals.

The same principles later powered **mRNA vaccines,** which use lipid nanoparticles (LNPs) to deliver fragile RNA strands into cells—another chapter in the liposome's long journey from the microscope slides of Cambridge to the frontlines of global health.

Today, when we design a new liposomal supplement, cosmetic, or drug, we are standing on the shoulders of that first success story. Doxil wasn't just a product; it was a **proof of concept** for the idea that *a drug's true potential lies in its delivery.*

9.9. Epilogue

When the FDA granted Doxil approval in 1995, it marked more than a regulatory milestone—it marked the moment when a scientific curiosity became a life-saving technology.

From Bangham's simple lecithin bubbles to a billion-dollar therapeutic class, the liposome had come full circle—a testament to how **a tiny bubble, when engineered with purpose, can carry not just medicine, but hope.**

Chapter 10

Relevance in Nutraceutical and Topical Liposomes

In nutraceutical applications, most formulations are designed to stay **fluid at room and body temperature** to ensure instant dispersion and absorption. For this reason, sunflower PC, soy PC, and egg PC—all of which have low or negative T_m—are ideal. These remain in the liquid-crystalline phase at all physiological temperatures, ensuring that nutrients like **vitamin C, quercetin, or CoQ10** are rapidly bioavailable.

In topical systems, however, a slightly higher T_m can be beneficial because it provides viscosity and structural stability in creams and gels. Liposomes with a T_m near **35–40 °C** stay semi-rigid at room temperature (improving texture) but become fluid on contact with warm skin, releasing the active precisely when applied.

That's why formulations for **niosomal or liposomal serums** often balance lipids of different chain lengths—creating a smooth transition that mimics the skin's own thermodynamic behavior.

10.1. T_m and the Future of Liposome Engineering

Today, we can measure and manipulate T_m with molecular precision. Advanced computational models and **molecular dynamics simulations** predict how a change in lipid type shifts the transition. This allows formulation scientists to design liposomes that "wake up" at specific body regions or external triggers.

We now see **pH- and temperature-dual responsive systems**, where the T_m is intentionally set near 37 °C but can be fine-tuned by local acidity. For example, in an inflamed intestine, where pH drops and tissue temperature rises slightly, such a liposome would cross its T_m threshold—becoming fluid, merging with membranes, and releasing the encapsulated antioxidant or peptide exactly where needed.

In the nutraceutical world, we don't yet use thermal targeting, but the same principle helps us **stabilize powders and beadlets.** When a Metazome® beadlet is stored below the lipid's T_m, the bilayer remains in the gel state—immobile, stable, and resistant to oxidation. When the consumer rehydrates it in water, the temperature instantly moves above T_m, re-fluidizing the membrane so it reforms nanosized liposomes in seconds. The system, in effect, "wakes up."

10.2. The Breathing Threshold of Life

In a poetic sense, T_m is the liposome's *breathing threshold.* Below it, the vesicle is asleep—rigid, silent, preserved.

Above it, it awakens into motion—dynamic, flexible, responsive. Every living membrane in nature has its own T_m, fine-tuned by evolution so that at body temperature it is neither too rigid nor too leaky.

When we design liposomes, we are essentially recapitulating that evolutionary trick: choosing lipids whose phase transition matches our purpose, whether that's long-term storage, gentle release, or triggered activation.

The next time you see a liposome under the microscope, imagine this invisible moment—the temperature where molecules start to dance, the structure expands, and the membrane begins to breathe. That is $\mathbf{T_m}$—the delicate line between stillness and life.

Chapter

11

Phosphatidylcholine – The Brick of the Bubble

Every liposome begins with a single, elegant molecule—**phosphatidylcholine**, or simply **PC**.

If you imagine a liposome as a tiny soap bubble, PC is the *soap*. It's the molecule that knows how to live in two worlds at once—the watery world and the oily one.

Chemically, PC looks like a **two-tailed tadpole**:

- The *head* is **hydrophilic** (water-loving)—it contains a phosphate group and choline, both charged and happy to face water.
- The *tails* are **hydrophobic** (water-hating) fatty acids—they avoid water and prefer to hide with other lipids.

When PC molecules are dropped into water, they instantly start self-organizing—because every part of the molecule wants to be somewhere specific. The heads rush toward water; the tails run away from it. This tension creates **self-assembly**, nature's way of building walls without any tools.

11.1. Why Phosphatidylcholine Is So Special

There are many phospholipids in biology—phosphatidylethanolamine, phosphatidylserine, phosphatidylglycerol—but **PC is the most balanced one**.

Its molecular shape is like a **cylinder**, not a cone.

That means the cross-sectional area of its head and its tails are roughly equal.

This geometry naturally favors **flat or gently curved bilayers**—perfect for forming the walls of liposomes and cell membranes.

Because PC is **zwitterionic** (it has both a positive and a negative charge but is overall neutral), it doesn't repel neighboring molecules strongly. Instead, it packs neatly with others, forming smooth, stable films.

That's why, in almost every liposome recipe, you'll see **50% or more PC**.

It forms the structural backbone—the stable matrix—while other lipids fine-tune properties like flexibility, charge, and permeability.

11.2. How It Curves to Make a Sphere

Imagine, for a moment, a vast microscopic landscape—water stretching endlessly in all directions. Into this world enters a population of molecules with a peculiar duality: phosphatidylcholine, often abbreviated as PC. Each molecule carries within it a quiet contradiction.

One end—the head—is drawn to water, almost eager to interact, to dissolve, to belong. The other end—the tail—is deeply averse, recoiling from water as if from an unseen threat.

When dispersed in water, these molecules do not remain scattered for long. There is an immediate, almost instinctive reorganization. The hydrophilic heads orient themselves toward the surrounding water, while the hydrophobic tails retreat from it. The result is not random clustering, but order—precise, repeating, and remarkably elegant.

They assemble into a sheet.

In this sheet, the tails hide inward, shielded from water, while the heads face outward on both sides, interacting comfortably with the aqueous environment. This is the bilayer—the same fundamental architecture that defines every living cell, every organelle, every boundary that separates life from its surroundings.

At first glance, the bilayer appears stable, almost complete. But at its edges lies a problem—one that the system cannot ignore.

Along the edges of this sheet, the hydrophobic tails are exposed. They face the very environment they are designed to avoid. This exposure is energetically unfavorable. Water molecules, highly structured and dynamic, resist accommodating these hydrophobic regions. The system, therefore, is under tension—not mechanical tension, but thermodynamic tension. It seeks a configuration of lower energy, of greater stability.

And so, the sheet begins to change.

Not abruptly, not through any external command, but through a gradual, collective response. The edges start to curve inward. The structure bends, folds, and reshapes itself. Every movement is guided by the same principle: minimize exposure of the hydrophobic tails to water.

As the curvature increases, the edges approach each other. Eventually, they meet—and when they do, the sheet closes upon itself.

What was once a flat plane becomes a sphere.

This transformation is profound. The exposed edges disappear. The hydrophobic tails are now completely hidden within the interior of the membrane, safely sandwiched between layers of hydrophilic heads. The system has reached a new equilibrium—a state where unfavorable interactions are minimized, and stability is maximized.

The result is a liposome.

A tiny, spherical vesicle with a hollow aqueous core, enclosed by a bilayer shell. Inside, water is trapped. Outside, water surrounds it. Between these two aqueous worlds lies a thin, ordered membrane—only a few nanometers thick—yet structurally robust and dynamically alive.

This entire process unfolds without guidance, without machinery, without energy input in the conventional sense. It is driven by fundamental physical forces: hydrophobic interactions, van der Waals forces, entropy, and the relentless tendency of systems to move toward lower free energy.

It is, in essence, self-organization.

But calling it merely "self-assembly" understates its elegance. This is molecular choreography—countless molecules moving in concert, each responding to its local environment, yet collectively producing a structure of remarkable precision and function.

The liposome is not just a structure; it is a solution. A resolution to the conflict between water-loving heads and water-fearing tails. A compromise that satisfies both, without sacrificing either.

And in this quiet transformation—from sheet to sphere—lies one of the most fundamental principles of life itself: that complexity need not be imposed from outside. It can emerge, naturally and inevitably, from the intrinsic properties of matter.

No external force. No guiding hand.

Just molecules, water, and the physics of belonging.

11.3. Why About 50% PC?

When scientists make liposomes, PC provides the right balance between **rigidity and flexibility**.

- If you use **too little PC**, the bilayer becomes unstable or leaky.
- If you use **too much PC**, it can get too fluid and fragile.
- Around **50% PC** (with the rest being helper lipids like phosphatidylethanolamine, sphingomyelin, or stabilizers like cholesterol) gives you **optimal packing**: strong enough to hold together, but flexible enough to curve naturally into spheres.

This ratio also mimics biological membranes—your own cell membranes are roughly 40–50% phosphatidylcholine by composition. Nature, too, has settled on the same formula.

11.4. The Curvature Story in Visual Terms

Let's translate geometry into imagery.

Lipid shape	Example lipid	Behavior in water	Structure formed
Cone-shaped (large head, short tails)	Lysophospha-tidylcholine	Curves outward	Micelles (single layer spheres)
Cylinder-shaped (balanced head & tails)	Phosphatidy-lcholine	Flat → gently curves	Bilayers → Liposomes
Inverted cone-shaped (small head, bulky tails)	Phosphatidy-lethanolamine	Curves inward	Inverted hexagonal phases

PC sits right in the **middle zone**—its cylindrical geometry makes it perfect for wrapping into closed vesicles without creating tension or collapse.

When energy is added (like mild heating or hydration), the PC molecules gain mobility. The bilayer undulates, bends, and finally closes into a sphere to eliminate edge exposure—the most energy-efficient configuration possible.

That's why PC-based liposomes are **spontaneously self-forming**—no complicated chemistry needed.

Chapter 12

From Sunflower to Science

In modern formulations, most PC comes from **soy lecithin** or **sunflower lecithin**. These natural sources yield **phosphatidylcholine-rich fractions** that are purified and standardized.

Sunflower PC has an added advantage—it's **non-GMO, plant-based, allergen-free**, and contains a balanced ratio of unsaturated fatty acids (like oleic and linoleic acid). These fatty acids make the membrane more fluid and flexible—an essential property for liposomes meant to survive processing, drying, and digestion.

So when you see "Sunflower PC 50%" in a liposome recipe, it's not an arbitrary choice—it's the **molecular blueprint of stability and elegance.**

12.1. A Simple Analogy

If a liposome were a house:

- **Phosphatidylcholine** is the brick—it forms the structure.
- **Cholesterol** is the cement—it fills the tiny gaps and gives strength.

- **Water** is the space inside—the room where the medicine lives.

Together, they build a structure that's both solid and dynamic—strong enough to survive the journey, yet flexible enough to merge with living cells.

12.2. In One Sentence

Phosphatidylcholine is the **architect of the liposome**.

Its balanced shape, dual-loving nature, and self-organizing behavior make it nature's most perfect molecule for building microscopic spheres of life.

12.2.1. Water's Personality—A Polar Molecule with Rules

Water molecules are like tiny magnets: one side slightly positive (hydrogen atoms), the other slightly negative (oxygen).

They **love order**—they cling to each other through hydrogen bonds, forming a constantly shifting but structured network.

But when a **non-polar molecule** like a fatty acid tail appears, water faces a dilemma—it can't form hydrogen bonds with it. That disrupts water's orderly network, creating "chaos" around the hydrophobic surface.

To restore order, water does something clever—it **forces those non-polar tails to huddle together**, minimizing their contact with water.

This is called the **hydrophobic effect**, and it's the single most powerful force behind the existence of membranes, micelles, and liposomes.

12.2.2. The Self-Assembly—How Water Orchestrates Structure

When phosphatidylcholine molecules are placed in water, two things happen instantly:

- Their **hydrophilic heads** (with phosphate and choline) reach out to bond with water molecules through electrostatic and hydrogen-bond interactions.
- Their **hydrophobic tails** (fatty acid chains) recoil from water, clustering together.

To satisfy both desires, the PC molecules **self-organize** into a **bilayer sheet**—heads facing the water on both sides, tails hidden inside, sandwiched between them.

But this sheet has a problem: its **edges expose hydrophobic tails to water**, which water absolutely hates.

The simplest way to eliminate those exposed edges?

Bend the sheet.

And the most efficient way to eliminate edges completely?

Close it into a sphere.

The sphere—a liposome—is nature's way of saying:

"No hydrophobic tail shall touch me!"

12.2.3. Why a Sphere, and Not a Cube or Cylinder?

Water always seeks the **lowest-energy configuration**—the arrangement that requires the least disturbance to its own structure.

A **sphere** gives the **maximum volume with the least surface area**, meaning fewer exposed edges, less interfacial tension, and a more stable system.

In the bilayer, every PC molecule can keep its head in contact with water while the tails stay safely buried. The curvature distributes mechanical stress evenly, creating a stable, flexible, self-healing structure.

That's why **a flat sheet curves into a bubble**, not a box or a sheet of wrinkles.

The geometry of curvature is dictated by water's energetic demand for **minimal disruption**—and PC's perfect cylindrical shape allows that curvature to occur smoothly.

12.2.4. The Water Inside—Not Just Filler, But Function

The water **trapped inside** the liposome's hollow core is not accidental. It's essential.

(a) It defines the liposome's identity

The presence of an internal aqueous compartment distinguishes **liposomes** from simple emulsions or oil droplets.

It means the liposome can carry **both water-soluble (hydrophilic)** and **fat-soluble (hydrophobic)** molecules at once:

- Water-soluble actives stay **inside** the aqueous core.
- Fat-soluble actives embed **within the bilayer membrane**.

That dual-compartment property is what makes liposomes truly multifunctional carriers.

(b) It stabilizes the bilayer

The water inside pushes gently outward, balancing the tension of the lipid layer.

It hydrates the polar head groups, keeps them spaced at optimal distance, and prevents collapse of the vesicle.

Without the internal water, the bilayer would stick together and form a dense, waxy mass—like dehydrated fat rather than a dynamic, living vesicle.

(c) It allows flexibility and fusion

A hydrated liposome is fluid and mobile.

The inner and outer water layers act like lubricants, letting liposomes deform, merge, and recover—behaviors essential for delivery through biological membranes.

12.2.5. When Water Creates Life-Like Behavior

In many ways, liposomes mimic **cells**, and that's no coincidence—the first biological membranes formed in the same way, billions of years ago.

When primitive fatty acids encountered early oceans, water's polarity drove them to self-assemble into microscopic spheres—protocells, capable of separating "inside" from "outside."

That was the birth of compartmentalized chemistry—and eventually, life itself.

Even today, when we make liposomes in the lab, we are **replaying nature's earliest act of self-organization**:

Lipid meets water → tension arises → structure forms → order emerges.

Water, through its quiet insistence on order, becomes the sculptor of biology.

12.2.6. The Dance Between Water and Lipid

You can imagine this like a dance:

- Water pulls the polar heads outward, whispering "face me."
- Lipid tails pull inward, saying "hide me."
- The compromise between the two is a **bilayer bubble**, curved and sealed, where both can coexist peacefully.

It's not chemistry alone—it's **thermodynamic diplomacy**.

Chapter 13

The Future of Liposomes in Supplements – Science, Standards, and Real-World Use

The supplement aisle is no longer defined by loud claims and striking labels. A quieter transformation is underway—one driven by engineering at the molecular scale. The true innovation now resides within the capsule, in structures designed to behave with the precision of biological systems. At the center of this evolution is the liposome.

Liposomes first proved their worth in medicine, where they demonstrated an ability to protect delicate molecules, navigate complex biological environments, and release actives with controlled precision. When this concept transitions into nutrition, the same scientific principles apply, but the context changes. Supplements must coexist with food, maintain palatability, remain stable over long shelf lives, and comply with regulatory frameworks that emphasize safety and cautious communication. Designing an effective liposomal supplement, therefore, becomes an exercise in integration—uniting membrane biophysics, food science, and human behavior into a single system.

A genuine liposome is a closed bilayer vesicle—an organized, spherical structure formed by phospholipids in water. This distinction is fundamental. It is not a micelle, which consists of a single-layer arrangement lacking an internal aqueous space. It is not a nanoemulsion, where oil droplets are stabilized by surfactants. Nor is it a simple dispersion of phospholipids without structural integrity. A true liposome offers two functional compartments at once: an aqueous interior capable of encapsulating hydrophilic molecules and a lipid bilayer that accommodates hydrophobic compounds. This dual architecture enables simultaneous delivery of chemically diverse actives within a single system.

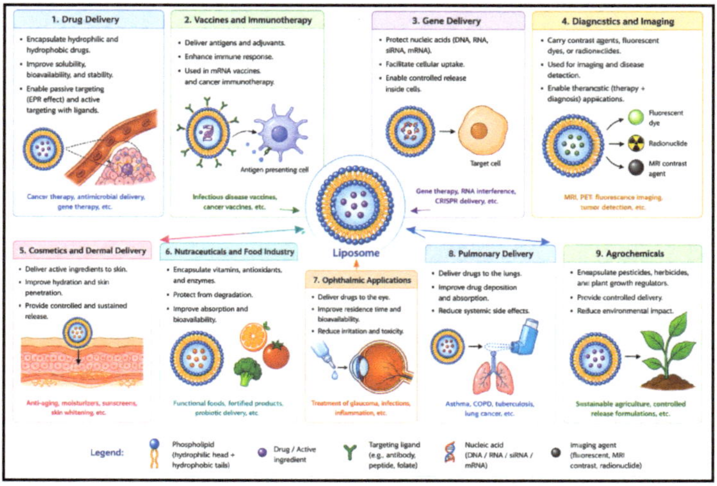

Figure 12. Applications of liposomes.

Schematic illustration of the diverse applications of liposomes, including drug delivery, vaccines and immunotherapy, gene delivery, diagnostics and imaging, cosmetics and dermal delivery, nutraceuticals, ophthalmic applications, pulmonary delivery, and agrochemical uses. These applications leverage the ability of liposomes to encapsulate bioactive compounds, enhance stability and bioavailability, and enable targeted and controlled delivery.

Verification of such structures requires rigorous characterization. Particle size and distribution are assessed through dynamic light scattering. Surface behavior is evaluated using zeta potential. The defining bilayer is visualized with cryogenic transmission electron microscopy. Most critically, analytical methods must confirm true encapsulation by distinguishing between free and entrapped actives. Structural integrity alone is not sufficient. Functional performance must also be demonstrated. When exposed to simulated digestive conditions, well-designed liposomes maintain stability long enough to reach the small intestine. Systems that disintegrate immediately under bile salt conditions fail to meet this standard. Phosphatidylcholine derived from sunflower serves as an effective membrane-forming lipid, enabling stable and tightly packed bilayers without the necessity of cholesterol when appropriately engineered.

The journey of an oral supplement is complex. It begins in the acidic environment of the stomach, progresses through enzymatic digestion in the intestine, and encounters bile salts that actively reorganize lipids. Beyond this lies the mucus barrier and the selective uptake mechanisms of intestinal cells. Phosphatidylcholine integrates naturally into this environment, participating in mixed micelle formation, interacting dynamically with biological membranes, and following metabolic pathways similar to dietary lipids. Properly engineered liposomes, typically within the nanoscale range, persist long enough to reach the small intestine, where interaction with bile components and cellular structures begins. Hydrophilic actives may be released in proximity to the intestinal lining, enabling diffusion or transport into cells, while hydrophobic molecules associate with cellular membranes and enter lipid-processing pathways within enterocytes. From there, incorporation into chylomicrons enables transport via the lymphatic system, allowing partial bypass of hepatic first-pass metabolism and often resulting in improved systemic exposure.

Effective liposomal design begins with the intrinsic properties of the active compound. Hydrophilic molecules require maximization of internal aqueous volume and strategies that minimize leakage. Lipophilic compounds demand a bilayer environment that promotes strong partitioning and prevents crystallization or expulsion. For ionizable molecules, engineered gradients between the interior and exterior of the vesicle can facilitate efficient loading and retention. Across these variations, the phospholipid membrane remains the central structural element, providing stability and functionality through precise control of composition and process.

Traditional liposomal supplements were predominantly liquid formulations. While functional, they presented limitations such as susceptibility to oxidation, strong taste profiles, and challenges in storage and transport. The transition to solid-state liposomes represents a significant advancement. In this form, liposomal structures are embedded within powders, granules, or beadlets that reconstruct into nanoscale vesicles upon hydration. Achieving this requires preservation of the bilayer's structural integrity during drying, protection of membrane spacing and hydration characteristics, and control of oxidative stability. Upon rehydration, the system must reliably reproduce the original vesicle size and distribution. When executed effectively, solid liposomes retain the functional benefits of liquid systems while offering enhanced stability, convenience, and scalability.

Scientific validation is essential to distinguish functional systems from superficial claims. A structured approach to evidence spans simulated digestion models that evaluate behavior under physiological conditions, cellular systems that assess transport potential, ex vivo tissues that reveal absorption pathways, and human pharmacokinetic studies that confirm systemic exposure. Parameters such as area under the curve, peak concentration, and time to peak provide quantitative measures of performance, while validated biomarkers offer insight where direct measurement is challenging. This continuum—from mechanism to human data—forms the foundation of credible liposomal science.

Supplements are consumed within the complexity of daily life, and food interactions cannot be ignored. Dietary fats can enhance bile secretion and support the uptake of lipid-associated actives, while other dietary components may compete for transport pathways or influence stability. Formulation characteristics such as pH, osmolality, and viscosity affect both sensory perception and gastrointestinal transit. Designing with these factors in mind ensures consistent performance beyond controlled laboratory conditions.

The effectiveness of a liposomal supplement must persist throughout its shelf life. Stability extends beyond initial characterization to long-term performance, requiring monitoring of particle size, distribution, surface charge, encapsulation efficiency, and chemical integrity. Oxidative markers, moisture content, and microbial limits must remain within defined boundaries. Packaging systems incorporating high-barrier materials, controlled atmospheres, and moisture management play a critical role in preserving product integrity. The objective is consistency, ensuring that the formulation performs identically from production to consumption.

Certain classes of compounds derive particular benefit from liposomal delivery, especially those that are fragile, poorly absorbed, or subject to significant first-pass metabolism. In these cases, the liposome functions not merely as a carrier but as an enabling system that transforms the pharmacokinetic profile of the active compound.

Within the supplement industry, regulatory frameworks require careful communication. Claims must emphasize support and maintenance rather than treatment, and all statements must be grounded in verifiable evidence. Transparency in formulation and mechanism bridges the gap between complex science and consumer understanding, ensuring responsible innovation.

Scaling liposomal systems from laboratory to manufacturing demands precision. Controlled processing techniques ensure consistent particle size and distribution, while drying technologies for solid systems must preserve structural integrity without introducing instability. Process monitoring and release testing are aligned with real-world use conditions to ensure that performance in the consumer's hands reflects laboratory characterization.

The future of liposomal supplements lies in refinement and personalization. Advances in computational modeling, biological understanding, and manufacturing flexibility will enable tailored delivery systems that align with individual physiology and lifestyle. Combinations of actives, targeted release mechanisms, and intelligent membrane designs will expand the capabilities of this platform.

At its core, liposomal delivery succeeds by aligning with biological principles rather than opposing them. A phospholipid membrane, engineered with precision and validated through rigorous science, mirrors the fundamental architecture of living systems. When consistently executed, liposomal technology moves beyond marketing language and becomes what it was always meant to be—a reliable, scientifically grounded method for delivering nutrition with the elegance and intelligence of a living cell.

Top of Form

Bottom of Form

in with, or they were poorly engineered. My formulations use **sunflower phosphatidylcholine (PC)** as the primary membrane former, and—by design—**do not require cholesterol**. With the right lipid architecture and process, the membrane can be tight, stable, and reproducible without it.

13.1. How a liposomal supplement navigates the gut.

Oral delivery is a long journey: acid in the stomach, enzymes in the small intestine, bile salts that form mixed micelles, a mucus barrier, and finally the enterocytes and M-cells that decide what gets in. Phosphatidylcholine is a native citizen in this environment; it blends into mixed micelles, fuses and exchanges lipids with membranes, and is metabolized like dietary fat. Properly sized vesicles—typically near the one-hundred-nanometer mark—survive long enough to reach the small intestine, where some fraction reorganizes with bile components and some fraction interacts directly with the intestinal lining. Hydrophilic payloads can be released near the membrane to diffuse or be transported inward; hydrophobic payloads partition into the enterocyte membrane and hitch a ride into chylomicron assembly. That last pathway is important: when an active enters via the lymph rather than the portal vein, it can partially bypass the liver's first-pass metabolism and show a higher **AUC** and **Cmax** in plasma. This is one scientific reason properly designed liposomes can outperform conventional powders for compounds like **curcumin, quercetin, resveratrol, CoQ10, PEA, black-ginger methoxyflavones, and reduced glutathione**.

13.2. Designing for the molecule, not forcing the molecule to fit.

The membrane recipe follows the payload. For water-soluble actives such as **vitamin C** or **glutathione**, I maximize aqueous entrapment with vesicle geometry and process conditions that increase internal water volume and limit leak. For oil-soluble actives such as **curcumin, CoQ10, black-ginger actives, and silymarin**, I tune the bilayer so the drug partitions strongly into the membrane and doesn't recrystallize. For weak acids and bases (for example, **berberine** in our advanced systems), I create internal–external gradients that "pull" the molecule into the vesicle after it forms and keep it there. All of this is done with **sunflower PC** as the membrane backbone, and without the need for cholesterol.

13.3. Liquid vs. solid – why dry liposomes change the category.

Classical liposomal supplements were liquids in bottles. They worked, but they tasted strong, oxidized faster, and were hard to ship. The major advance is making **true liposomes as solids**—powders, granules, beadlets, even **chewables**—that spring back into nanoscale vesicles the moment water hits them. I developed **Metazome®** precisely for this: a solid-state architecture built around sunflower PC that preserves bilayer integrity during drying, storage, and even compression. In practice this means I can put a liposomal vitamin C or a liposomal black-ginger extract into a capsule, a stick pack, or a tablet, with a shelf life measured in years, not weeks. The science behind that is straightforward to state and hard to execute: you must protect the bilayer's spacing and hydration shell in the dry state (we use specific sugars and processing profiles), prevent oxidative attack (choose low-peroxide excipients and high-barrier packaging), and ensure that rehydration reconstructs the same size and dispersion we made on day one. When you get those three right, solid liposomes behave like their liquid cousins—without the headaches.

Chapter

14

Evidence that Convinces Scientists and Regulators.

Supplements are not drugs, but evidence still matters. I build dossiers in layers. First, **in-vitro digestion** using the international INFOGEST protocol tells me how the vesicles behave under gastric and intestinal conditions. Then **Caco-2** monolayers or intestinal organoids indicate whether we improved transepithelial transport. **Ex vivo** intestinal tissues can show uptake pathways. Finally, **human PK**—properly randomized, crossover, fed vs. fasted—answers the only question consumers and physicians ask: does more of the active reach the blood, and how fast? I measure **AUC**, **Cmax**, and **Tmax**, and for actives with difficult plasma analytics I use validated biomarkers (for example, **reduced glutathione** levels, **oxidative-stress panels**, **NO-related flow measures** for black-ginger). Where appropriate, I add **PBPK modeling** to explain why the profile improves (for example, higher lymphatic contribution or reduced presystemic metabolism). That scientific arc—mechanism, model, human PK—separates real liposomes from marketing mirages.

14.1. Formulation meets food – the matrix effect is real.

Supplements are taken with meals, coffee, protein shakes, and sometimes nothing at all. Fat in the meal amplifies bile release and can help liposomal uptake of lipophobes; polyphenol-rich foods can compete for transporters; calcium can complex certain actives. I design dosing instructions around those facts. For membrane-loving actives, "with a main meal" is often best; for hydrophiles that diffuse independently, timing is more flexible. Osmolality, pH, and viscosity of the finished product affect gastric emptying and taste; I keep osmolality moderate and avoid aggressive solvents so that the sensory profile is clean even in **ready-to-mix** sticks and **RTD** beverages.

14.2. Quality that lasts the whole shelf life.

A liposomal supplement is only as good as day-720 data. I work to **ICH**-style stability: long-term and accelerated conditions with periodic checks of size, polydispersity, zeta potential, potency, encapsulation, oxidation markers (peroxide value, p-anisidine), moisture and water activity for solids, and microbial limits. For powders and beadlets I choose high-barrier laminates, nitrogen flush, desiccants where appropriate, and headspace oxygen targets. For flavor systems I prefer natural complexes that don't attack the membrane. Every decision is pointed at one outcome: when the consumer opens the pack months later, the vesicles they ingest behave like the ones I characterized in the lab.

14.3. Where liposomes make the biggest difference today.

Some actives are natural fits. **Vitamin C** benefits from protection and gentler gastric experience. **Reduced glutathione** is fragile and oxidizes; the bilayer shields it. **CoQ10** and **curcumin** are classic lipophobes with low baseline absorption; the membrane pathway and lymphatic entry help them. **Berberine** faces first-pass metabolism; a liposomal approach can alter exposure profiles while preserving tolerability. **Black-ginger methoxyflavones** pair beautifully with membranes and show vascular and performance support endpoints that are measurable within weeks. Minerals are more nuanced: while ionic species don't "live" in a bilayer, a well-designed liposomal powder can co-deliver chelates or organo-salts with membrane support for comfort and kinetics.

14.4. Regulatory reality and responsible claims.

In the United States, supplements must be **safe**, **truthful in labeling**, and limited to **structure/function** claims (no disease claims). Europe is even stricter on claims; India aligns safety first. I avoid the word "treat," use measured language—"supports," "helps maintain," "promotes"—and I tie every statement to data I can show. I also define "liposome" in consumer-friendly words on pack and back it with a one-page technical brief. That transparency is good science and good business.

14.5. Manufacturing that scales without losing the nanoscale.

At pilot and commercial scale I prefer **microfluidic or controlled-shear solvent-dilution** to get tight size and narrow distributions, followed by **tangential-flow filtration** to exchange solvents and set the final buffer. For solid forms, I use **lyophilization** or gentle **spray drying** into carriers that protect the bilayer and enable **Metazome®** beadlet architecture. Throughout, process analytical tools track particle size in-line, and release testing reflects how the consumer will actually use the product (for example, reconstitution in 200–250 mL water, then immediate simulated-digestion challenge).

14.6. Where this is going next.

The near future is personalization and combinations. One can imagine AI-guided selection of dose and format based on genotype, microbiome, and lifestyle, then manufacturing **on demand**—solid liposomes that carry a **hydrophile in the core** and a **lipophile in the membrane**, released differentially across the gut. I see intelligent coatings that sense pH and bile patterns to time opening, and membranes that carry tiny targeting ligands for specific epithelial pathways without sacrificing safety. Most importantly, I see the category maturing: fewer "liposomal" labels on products that aren't, and more rigorous science on products that are.

In short, liposomal supplements succeed when they act like biology rather than fight it. A membrane made from **sunflower PC**, engineered **without cholesterol**, assembled with precision, proven in digestion models and humans, and stabilized as a **solid that rehydrates to the same nanoscale vesicles**—this is not a marketing story; it is a manufacturing discipline. Do that consistently, and "liposomal" stops being a buzzword and becomes what it should be: a reliable way to deliver nutrition with the grace and intelligence of a living cell.

Chapter

15

Forgotten Pioneers and Stories

Every scientific breakthrough hides a trail of forgotten names—people whose work quietly built the staircase others climbed. The story of liposomes is no exception. We often remember Alec Bangham as the father of liposomes, but like any great discovery, it was born in collaboration, curiosity, and even coincidence.

When you trace back the roots of liposomal science, you find an intriguing web of ideas stretching across centuries—from Mendeleev's musings on colloids to the flickering black-and-white images captured by a young electron microscopist named R. W. Horne.

15.1. R. W. Horne – The Man Behind the First Liposome Image

While Bangham provided the ideas, **R. W. Horne** provided the eyes. In the early 1960s, the electron microscope was a mysterious, almost magical instrument. Each image required days of sample preparation, ultra-thin sectioning, and metal shadowing techniques that demanded near-surgical precision.

Horne was a master of this craft. Working with Bangham at the Babraham Institute in Cambridge, he coated lipid films with a fine layer of **platinum** and recorded their images on glass photographic plates. What he saw were concentric circles—shimmering rings that looked like miniature onions. These weren't crystals or contaminants; they were **self-assembled lipid membranes** enclosing water.

Those photographs became the first visual evidence of what we now call **liposomes**. Without Horne's patient work and his pioneering mastery of electron microscopy, the phenomenon might have gone unnoticed, or dismissed as a strange artifact. In many ways, Horne was the **first to truly see life's architecture recreated outside of biology.**

Bangham once joked that Horne "made membranes speak." And indeed, those grainy platinum-coated pictures spoke louder than words—showing, for the first time, that life's defining boundary could be mimicked in the lab.

15.2. Mendeleev and the Colloidal Vision – An Idea Before Its Time

If we travel further back—more than 70 years before liposomes were discovered—we find **Dimitri Ivanovich Mendeleev**, best known as the creator of the periodic table. But Mendeleev was more than a chemist who organized elements; he was a philosopher of matter.

In **1889**, he wrote about **colloidal systems**—mixtures where substances neither dissolve completely nor separate, existing in a mysterious intermediate state. He speculated that in such systems, molecules might self-organize into ordered structures, forming "dynamic boundaries" that could explain many of nature's behaviors.

He didn't use the word *lipid* or *membrane*—those concepts hadn't yet been formalized—but what he described sounds strikingly similar to the **self-assembly** behavior of phospholipids that forms liposomes.

It's poetic to think that decades before modern biophysics, Mendeleev was already imagining molecular communities forming boundaries and compartments—an intellectual ancestor of what Bangham and Horne would later witness through the lens of an electron microscope.

15.3. The World's First Artificial Cell

By **1965**, Bangham's team at Cambridge had refined their techniques enough to present something truly extraordinary. They demonstrated that these lipid vesicles could **mimic biological cell membranes**—selectively allowing certain molecules to pass through while keeping others out.

In scientific circles, this was electrifying. For the first time, researchers had a **model system** to study the fundamental behavior of cell membranes outside living organisms. It was as if someone had taken the concept of "life's envelope" and reassembled it from scratch.

Bangham called it the **"phospholipid bilayer model"**, but to many others, it was more than that. Scientists around the world began referring to liposomes as the **"first artificial cells."**

This idea connected the discovery of liposomes to one of science's oldest questions—*how did life begin?*

If simple lipid molecules could spontaneously form closed vesicles in water, enclosing small molecules inside, could that have been how the **first protocells** appeared billions of years ago on the early Earth? In that sense, liposomes weren't just a tool for drug delivery—they were a glimpse into life's own origin story.

Even today, origin-of-life researchers create liposomes under simulated prebiotic conditions to explore how membranes might have formed spontaneously in ancient oceans. The same tiny bubbles that carry vitamins or cancer drugs today could once have been nature's first biological experiments.

15.4. The Forgotten Lab at Babraham

The Babraham Institute, where these discoveries unfolded, was not a glamorous research palace but a quiet countryside lab outside Cambridge, surrounded by green fields and the occasional sheep. In the early 1960s, it was far removed from the city's academic elite—a place where curiosity was allowed to wander freely.

Alec Bangham was known for his dry humor and modesty. He once said, *"We were simply trying to understand how membranes work. We didn't know we were inventing something."*

There's a beautiful irony there: while much of the world was racing toward nuclear physics and rockets, Bangham and Horne were quietly staring at bubbles—and found something equally powerful.

Their discovery didn't make headlines immediately. For nearly two decades, liposomes were more of a scientific curiosity than a commercial success. But when the first liposomal drug, **Doxil**, was approved in the 1990s, Bangham's work suddenly became legendary. It had taken over thirty years for the world to recognize the value of his small bubbles.

15.5. A Chain of Curiosity

Scientific discoveries rarely happen in isolation. They are chains of curiosity that stretch across generations. Mendeleev's vision of colloidal order in 1889 inspired the early colloid chemists of the 1930s. They, in turn, influenced Bangham's generation of membrane biophysicists. Bangham and Horne's work, initially inspired by the study of red blood cell membranes, created the foundation for liposomal drugs, vaccines, and even cosmetic serums.

It's humbling to realize that **one of the most advanced technologies of modern nanomedicine began as a simple observation of how lipids behave in water.**

The forgotten pioneers—Horne, Mendeleev, and countless unnamed lab assistants who pipetted, photographed, and theorized—each added a piece to this story. Science remembers the names on the papers, but history remembers the ones who *saw*.

15.6. A Poetic Legacy

In many ways, liposomes symbolize more than just scientific progress—they reflect humanity's deep fascination with **boundaries**. Every living thing, from a bacterium to a human brain cell, depends on a membrane that decides what enters and what stays out. To recreate that barrier in the laboratory is not just chemistry; it's philosophy in molecular form.

Bangham himself understood this. Late in life, he reflected on his discovery with characteristic understatement, saying, "*We were studying the skin of life, and accidentally made a living model of it.*"

That poetic statement still holds true. When we build liposomes today—whether to carry a cancer drug, a plant extract, or a vitamin—we are continuing that same experiment that began in Cambridge's quiet countryside. We are, in a way, still studying "the skin of life."

And in those shimmering, spherical bubbles, we can see both **the past and the future of biology**—from Mendeleev's vision of molecular order to the first artificial cells, and from the platinum-coated films of Horne's microscope to the advanced solid liposomes we design today.

The story of liposomes is not just about technology—it is about the people who dared to look closer at something as simple as fat and water and found, inside it, the essence of life itself.

Chapter

16

The Future of Liposomes: Where Chemistry Becomes Life

If there's one thing science teaches us, it's that big revolutions often come from the smallest places. The atom changed physics. The cell changed biology. And the liposome—a mere bubble a thousand times smaller than the width of a hair—is quietly changing the way we understand health, nutrition, and life itself.

This book began with a simple idea: how can we deliver a molecule to where it's needed most? Yet as we followed the story—from Alec Bangham's egg lecithin films to the advanced solid-state liposomes of today—we've realized something deeper. Liposomes are not just delivery systems. They are the language of living chemistry—a conversation between structure and function, matter and meaning.

16.1. The Bubble That Taught Us to Think

When Bangham looked through his electron microscope in the 1960s, he wasn't trying to invent a technology. He was trying to understand life's boundaries—the thin line that separates the inside from the outside, the self from the world. And what he found was something that behaves like life: it forms spontaneously, heals itself, and carries meaning in its structure.

In the decades that followed, liposomes moved from philosophical curiosity to pharmaceutical reality. They became the workhorses of modern drug delivery—carrying chemotherapy drugs, vaccines, antibiotics, and now even mRNA. Their story parallels humanity's greatest scientific transition—from chemistry to biology, and now to biotechnology.

But the story doesn't end there. Because now, liposomes have moved out of the hospital and into the kitchen, the cosmetic shelf, the nutraceutical factory, and even into outer space.

16.2. Liposomes in Daily Life

Look around. Liposomes are no longer confined to syringes or microscopes—they're in supplements, serums, and functional beverages. When you sip a liposomal vitamin drink, you are, without realizing it, consuming one of the most advanced biomimetic systems ever designed by science.

In skincare, liposomes carry plant actives deep into the epidermis, where creams once could never reach. They make antioxidants last longer, fragrances linger softer, and actives release smarter. In nutrition, they protect fragile vitamins like C, D, or K, and hydrophobic compounds like curcumin, CoQ10, and black-ginger flavones—helping them survive the stomach's harsh chemistry and slip into circulation seamlessly.

Even **NASA** has explored nanoencapsulation for long-duration missions, where radiation and oxidation threaten to destroy vitamins and lipids during space travel. Liposomes, with their double-layered shield, are logical candidates for **space nutrition**—microcosms of protection in the cosmic vacuum.

From the clinic to the cosmos, these tiny bubbles are expanding their influence like microscopic ambassadors of life.

16.3. When Nature Becomes the Teacher

What fascinates me most is how liposomes bring us closer to nature—not further from it.

We now know that plants release **exosome-like vesicles**, microscopic couriers that carry RNA and metabolites to communicate with other cells and even with the human gut microbiome. These natural nanocarriers are nature's version of liposomes—built from the same basic architecture, optimized by millions of years of evolution.

When we make liposomes from **sunflower phosphatidylcholine**, we're not inventing something foreign—we're continuing the conversation that leaves began billions of years ago. Our work is an extension of nature's design: refining it, stabilizing it, and guiding it for purpose.

The next time you drink orange juice or chew spinach, remember—you're consuming billions of natural nanovesicles that speak the same language as our engineered liposomes.

16.4. The Next Frontier –Smart, Personalized Liposomes

The liposomes of the future will be unrecognizable compared to the early lecithin vesicles of the 1960s. They will think, adapt, and respond. We are entering the age of **intelligent liposomes**.

- **Smart release systems** will sense pH, enzymes, or even body temperature, releasing nutrients only when and where needed.
- **AI-driven formulation** will design lipid compositions atom by atom, predicting stability, absorption, and bioavailability before the first batch is even mixed.
- **Personalized liposomes** will be tuned to each individual's microbiome, genetic profile, and metabolism—an intimate chemistry of one.
- **Hybrid liposomes** will merge biology and electronics—carrying magnetic or light-responsive nanoparticles that can be triggered externally.
- **Edible plant-derived vesicles** will blend into our food system—creating functional foods

that deliver actives as precisely as a medical injection, but as gently as a meal.

In essence, liposomes will become the **molecular interface between nutrition and medicine**—between food and therapy.

16.5. Solid-State and Beyond – The Engineering Evolution

For decades, one limitation of liposomes was fragility. They were like soap bubbles—beautiful, functional, but short-lived. Then came the revolution of **solid-state liposomes**—stable powders and beadlets that retain bilayer integrity even without water.

Technologies like **Metazome®**, born from our labs, are rewriting the rules: liposomes that can be compressed into chewables, packed into capsules, or even mixed into food matrices—then rehydrate back into nanosized vesicles in the body. These aren't just supplements; they are **living materials**—sleeping membranes that awaken in contact with water.

In the near future, such solid-state systems will underpin every advanced nutraceutical and cosmeceutical—from intelligent performance supplements to long-acting anti-aging formulations.

It's not science fiction. It's physics, chemistry, and life beautifully aligned.

16.6. Beyond the Body – Liposomes as Communicators

Liposomes are not only carriers of drugs or nutrients; they are communicators. Their very existence blurs the line between chemistry and biology. They respond to stimuli, sense their environment, self-heal, and even fuse with other membranes—behaviors we associate with living systems.

In synthetic biology, researchers are already using liposomes as **protocells**—simplified artificial cells that can carry enzymes, genetic material, and perform primitive metabolism. These experiments are part of the search for **the origin of life**. It's poetic to realize that the same structures we use for supplements might resemble the earliest ancestors of living cells on Earth.

What began as a delivery system may one day become a **platform for synthetic life**.

16.7. The Human Story

Science is rarely linear—it's full of detours, personalities, and poetic coincidences. Alec Bangham discovered liposomes in a countryside lab using egg yolk. Decades later, those same principles now power mRNA vaccines, advanced cancer therapies, and the nutraceuticals on your shelf.

It's also a story of persistence. For years, liposomes were dismissed as unstable, impractical, or too expensive. Today, they're the gold standard of encapsulation. The journey from Bangham's hand-cranked centrifuge to AI-optimized production lines is a testament to human curiosity—the one force as persistent as physics itself.

I often think of liposomes as a metaphor for science: fragile at first, misunderstood, but resilient enough to survive—and eventually, indispensable.

16.8. A Glimpse into Tomorrow

Picture a day not too far away:

Your breakfast smoothie contains personalized liposomal beadlets—each tuned for your age, metabolism, and genetic profile.

Your smartwatch tracks your nutritional levels in real time and communicates with a dispenser that releases the right liposomal nutrients on demand.

Your skincare cream contains hybrid liposomes that respond to UV exposure, releasing antioxidants exactly when your skin needs them.

Your functional food is no longer just nutrition—it's precision biochemistry woven into your daily routine.

And perhaps one day, liposomes will even help terraform life beyond Earth—delivering oxygen-generating enzymes or antioxidants to plants growing on Mars. The same bubble that once modeled the first cell on Earth might become the vessel of survival in space.

16.9. Epilogue – Small Bubbles, Endless Impact

When I look at a liposome under a microscope, I don't just see a vesicle.

I see a bridge—between biology and chemistry, nature and engineering, past and future.

Each one is a masterpiece of self-organization: a silent agreement among molecules to form order out of chaos. No human hand assembles them; they assemble themselves—as if the universe whispers, *"This is how life begins."*

From Bangham's thin lipid films observed under electron microscopy to AI-designed nanovesicles, from the human bloodstream to the silence of space—liposomes have shown us that the smallest systems often carry the largest meanings. They have reshaped medicine, empowered nutrition, revolutionized cosmetics, and ignited our imagination of life itself. So, when I say **"Small bubbles, big impact,"** I'm not describing a product.

I'm describing a philosophy—that in science, as in life, greatness often begins at the nanoscale.

The story of liposomes is far from over. In fact, it's only beginning.

The next generation of scientists and dreamers will write its next chapters—in clinics, kitchens, orbiting space stations, and perhaps even in the first living colonies on Mars.

And when they do, they will still be guided by the same principle that Bangham glimpsed six decades ago—that a simple bubble can hold not just a molecule, but **the idea of life itself**.

16.10. Author's Note – My Journey Inside the Bubble

My journey with liposomes began not in a factory or a corporate lab, but as a quiet fascination during my research years at **Deakin University in Australia**. I was drawn to the idea that a molecule could protect another molecule—that chemistry could be compassionate. Liposomes, to me, were more than nanocarriers; they were living metaphors of resilience, protection, and intelligence.

When I returned to India, this fascination transformed into purpose. Out of a modest setup with a handful of determined people, we built **Molecules Biolabs**—a science-first company with a dream far bigger than its size. From those early days of small mixers and sleepless nights to becoming one of India's most innovative liposomal technology groups, the journey has been humbling.

Then came **Akore Formulations**, born from a desire to take this science to the skin—to translate molecular precision into topical delivery. Akore became a bridge between advanced nanoscience and Ayurveda-inspired wellness, blending nature and nanotechnology into a single, coherent story.

And finally, **Atomins Innovations**—the new frontier. Conceived as the world's first **CRDMO for nutraceuticals**, Atomins represents not just the scaling of science, but the evolution of vision. It brings together artificial intelligence, formulation chemistry, and human curiosity into one collaborative ecosystem—from molecule to market, powered by science.

Each of these ventures is a reflection of the same principle that first fascinated me about liposomes—that great things are born when boundaries dissolve. Between chemistry and biology. Between nature and innovation. Between imagination and implementation.

As I look back, I realize that the story of liposomes and my own story are deeply intertwined—both began as fragile ideas, both faced skepticism, both found strength in structure and purpose.

From a student exploring molecular membranes at Deakin to the founder of a global family of scientific enterprises, this has been more than a professional journey—it has been a personal evolution.

If these pages have taught anything, I hope it is this:

That science, when pursued with conviction and creativity, can begin as a bubble in a beaker and end up touching lives across the world.

AI Usage Statement

Certain sections of this book have been refined for clarity and language using artificial intelligence (AI)-based tools, including ChatGPT. Additionally, selected schematic illustrations and figures have been generated or adapted with the assistance of AI technologies to enhance visual representation and understanding. All content has been carefully reviewed, edited, and validated by the author to ensure scientific accuracy and integrity.

www.ingramcontent.com/pod-product-compliance
Lightning Source LLC
LaVergne TN
LVHW051135210926
848482LV00006B/318

9798904513573